DAI MANUEL'S
WHOLE LIFE
FITNESS
MANIFESTO

DAI MANUEL'S
WHOLE LIFE FITNESS MANIFESTO

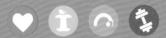

30 MINUTES A DAY FOR A HEALTHIER BODY, MIND AND SPIRIT

LifeTree
MEDIA

Cataloguing data available from Library and Archives Canada
ISBN 978-1-928055-07-5 (paperback)
ISBN 978-1-928055-08-2 (epub)
ISBN 978-1-928055-09-9 (pdf)

The information presented in this book is not intended as medical advice or as a substitute for medical counselling. Always consult your physician before beginning any exercise and nutrition program. If you choose not to obtain the consent of your physician and/or work with your physician throughout the duration of your time using the recommendations in this book you are agreeing to accept full responsibility for your actions and recognize that despite all precautions on the part of the author or publisher there are risks of injury or illness which can occur in connection with, or as a result of, use or misuse of the programs, exercises, advice, diets and/or information found in this book. You expressly assume such risks and waive, relinquish and release any claim which you may have against the author or publisher.

PUBLISHED BY
LifeTree Media Ltd.
www.lifetreemedia.com

DISTRIBUTED BY
Greystone Books Ltd.
www.greystonebooks.com

DISTRIBUTED IN THE U.S. BY
Publishers Group West

PHOTOGRAPHY BY Sombilon Photography, except for the following: Makito Inomata (Dai Manuel's quote sidebar "head" and page 168); Oren Jack Turner/Wikimedia Commons (page 11); A.F. Bradley/Wikimedia Commons (page 26); Mark Halliday (page 27, 154, 160 [bottom left], 161); National General Pictures/Wikimedia Commons (page 45); MetalGearLiquid/Wikimedia Commons (page 51); Soupstock/Bigstock.com (page 53); CBS Photo Archive (page 64); Purshi/Wikimedia Commons (page 65); Tenzin Choegyal (page 69); Matt Bevis (page 199 [left]); Brian Solis (page 120); Orange Memories Photography (page 157, 160 [top and bottom right], 174, 182 [top right]); and Associated Press (page 165). All testimonial photos are supplied courtesy of their subjects.

ILLUSTRATION BY Mauve Pagé, except Carolyn Lott (page 33); Hobbitfoot/Bigstock.com (page 67); Blackred/iStockphoto (page 79); Nuraschka/Bigstock.com.com (page 128) and Leontura/iStockphoto (page 164).

EDITING BY Lucy Hyslop and Maggie Langrick
COPYEDITING BY Rachel Eagen
DESIGN BY Mauve Pagé
PROOFREADING AND INDEX BY JoAnne Burek

PRINTED AND BOUND IN CANADA

To the women in my life, without you I never would have had the courage to write this book. To the men in my life, thank you for pushing me to never settle for anything less than I am capable of. And to everyone else...Hoorah!

I'm here to help people live happy, healthier, more active lifestyles while developing richer, deeper and more meaningful personal relationships with themselves, and their friends, families and communities.

CONTENTS

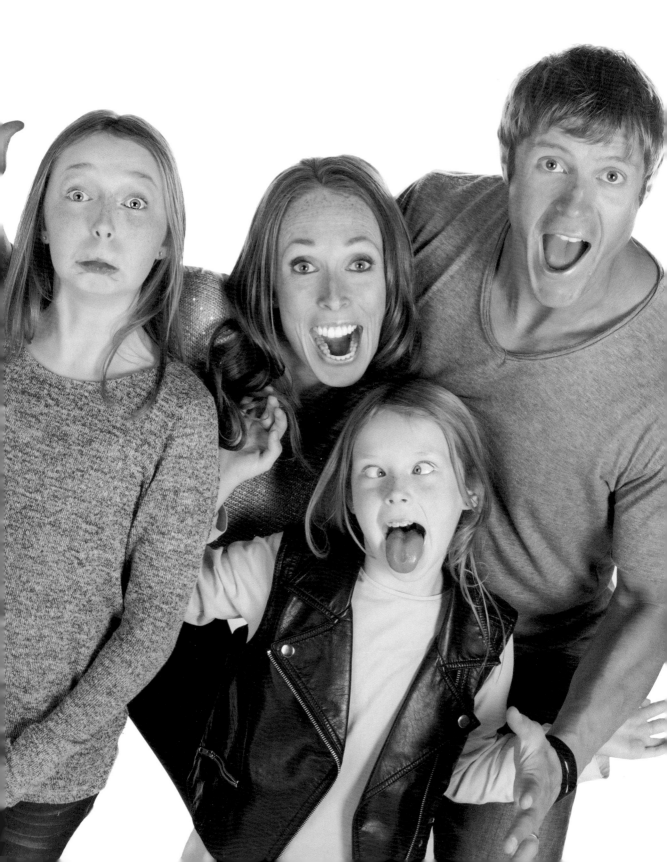

INTRODUCTION

DO YOU WANT TO LIVE a life of *total* awesomeness?

Some years ago, I asked myself that same question. I realized that while I had a lot to be thankful for in my life, I was falling short of my own potential. Don't get me wrong—I was doing the best I could, and life had been trucking along fine. I had moved to a new city on the West Coast, attended university, started to discover myself, landed a great job, fell in love, travelled a little and started a family. But I never seemed to have time for the things that were most important to me. I was also spending more money than I had.

My health and fitness ebbed and flowed throughout my life. When I only had to worry about myself, I could always find time for fitness. But when other people—my family—became a significant part of my life, I felt pulled to prioritize "us" rather than "me," and my health often suffered as a result. I figured that this was just the way it went; after all, it seemed like everyone else I knew was on the same path. But in the back of my mind, I was always thinking: *Is this* really *how life is supposed to be?*

As time went on, I kept trying to balance the priorities in my life, striving to attain "perfection," but I was constantly disappointed in myself. I was never able to truly balance it all. When I let one part of my life become the shining star, all other aspects of my life would dim in comparison. If I focused on family, my career suffered. When I turned my energies toward my career, in particular when I was building my company, my family felt it, and so did my health. I just never seemed to have enough to make everything work. Do you know the feeling?

Like many people, I found happy distraction in activities that didn't propel me forward in life—pub nights, boys' trips, nights out with my colleagues and long days on the golf course. I kept telling myself that tomorrow would be the day to "reset" and get everything in order: *Tomorrow is the day to start my new habits. Tomorrow is the start of my path to awesomeness.* But you know what? Every day I'd wake up to TODAY and TOMORROW would never arrive.

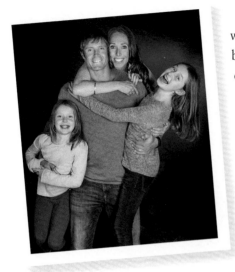

Me and the ladies in my life: Christie, Brielyn and Chardonae.

Maybe you can relate. Many of us put all of our obligations—whether it's work, family, or social life—ahead of our own well-being and personal growth. We're so busy taking care of what other people need from us that we forget to pay attention to our own needs. The problem with that is that while this might help us to get a lot done, mostly for others, we're probably not feeling satisfied with our lives. Even worse, if we're not careful, we can burn out—both mentally and physically. And when that happens, we not only let ourselves down, we also let down those who depend on us.

My goal in creating the *Whole Life Fitness Manifesto* is to sweep away the negative energies, accentuate the positive ones and empower YOU to radiate your own awesomeness, along with the greatness of those around you. In a nutshell, the *Whole Life Fitness Manifesto* is about putting yourself *first*, which will ultimately benefit those you care about. We all have people in our lives that matter to us. It's time we begin to matter to ourselves so that we can enjoy an incredible life with each other.

So, welcome to a new kind of fitness book. We're not just talking about physical fitness here. We're acknowledging that whole-life awesomeness encompasses fitness of mind, body and spirit. And because this is something that we all deserve, this book is for everyone. Even the most stamina-challenged person can tackle the Whole Life Fitness Power 30 program, which will also test you if you are already pushing your own fitness limits.

Getting a grip on total health and wellness is particularly important now because of disturbing rises in obesity and diabetes. Current health statistics, which you'll find throughout this book, are not pretty. In fact, they are a sobering wake-up call.

But there is reason for hope. On the other end of the spectrum, there is a booming personal growth movement, in which people are realizing their limitless potential as human beings. Put simply, linking your greater potential to your physical fitness is a powerful combination that can change—and possibly save—your life.

As you'll see, workouts don't have to be a chore. Working out is really about enjoying a burst of movement that can function as a reset, break, and check-in with your body throughout the day. It's about feeling how daily movement can activate all kinds of positive things in your life.

What makes me so certain about all this? Let me share a deeply personal story.

When I was a kid, there were two students in my school who were extremely overweight. I was one of them. As a 91-kg (200-lb) 15-year-old, I had a body mass index (BMI) of over 40; I was, by definition, *morbidly obese*. But after a big personal breakthrough shortly after my 15th birthday, I dug deep to make a change and, quite simply, I never looked back. My mental attitude played a pivotal role in making that change. I wanted to be healthy, happy and more satisfied with my life, and I did whatever it took to make that happen.

Today, I am honoured to be part of a healthy and beautiful family, with my wife, Christie, and my daughters, Chardonae and Brielyn. I constantly strive to live a life of which I'm proud. In my professional life, I've evolved from a successful fitness equipment entrepreneur to a personal trainer, lifestyle coach, speaker, author and all-around "life enhancer." I'm honoured to have the ability to help people every day—now that's pretty awesome!

Beyond my family, physical health and career, one of the most important aspects of my well-being is my mental health, or *emotional fitness*. I continually strive to cultivate a deep sense of purpose in my heart and mind; this is what makes me spring out of bed in the morning. And at the end of each day, I ask myself: *Was I the best person I could possibly be today?* If I can answer *yes* more often than not, then I know I'm on the right track.

I know we are all capable of achieving whole life fitness. That is, while I believe that we can work out on our own, we never have to *be* alone with our fitness and lifestyle goals. Now that you've found this book, you have found your community—your tribe. No matter what your current lifestyle, age, gender or personality, you are not alone. We are here to encourage and support each other to be the happiest, healthiest versions of ourselves.

So, hands up if you're ready for a whole life of awesomeness!

Dai Manuel
@DaiManuel

FEEL ENERGIZED

IF YOU DON'T **USE IT,** YOU **LOSE IT**

FOLLOW THE **5 Fs:**

FITNESS
FAMILY
FAITH
FINANCES
FUN!!

Tackle anything life throws at you— no matter how large the physical obstacle

THINK LESS OF AN **"I-WISH LIST"** AND MORE OF AN **"I-WILL LIST."**

HOW DO YOU WANT TO FEEL IN **10 20** OR **40?** YEARS

RECRUIT THE SAME MUSCLE GROUPS THAT ARE USED IN EVERYDAY REAL-LIFE SITUATIONS

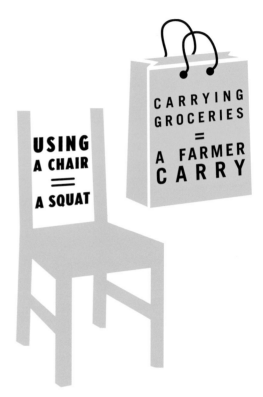

USING A CHAIR = A SQUAT

CARRYING GROCERIES = A FARMER CARRY

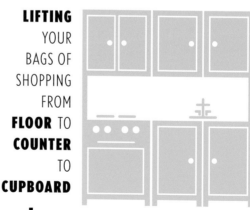

LIFTING YOUR BAGS OF SHOPPING FROM **FLOOR** TO **COUNTER** TO **CUPBOARD**

↳ **DEADLIFT + BICEP CURL + SHOULDER PRESS**

WHOLE LIFE FITNESS
CHAPTER 1

FITNESS IS BROKEN.

On any given day, the media would have us believe a range of wild claims: that a fat-reduced diet will make us skinny; that we can sculpt six-pack abs in three minutes or less; and that if we don't exercise for more than an hour a day, five days a week, we'll never reach our fitness goals. Above all, we are told that achieving a particular body shape will bring us happiness and fulfilment.

My answer to all this? *Garbage!*

Most people's beliefs around fitness are driven by vanities. Many of us feel pressure to attain a certain body type, or to achieve top athletic performance. Much of our framework is built on the preconceived notion that having a lean or muscular body is an indicator—the *only* indicator—of fitness. But appearances, however clichéd this may sound, really are only skin deep. Approach fitness in this way and you're following a Band-Aid approach to wellness that is simply unsustainable.

Over my nearly two decades in the health and fitness industry, I've seen my fair share of quick-fix thinking and short-term goal setting. Whether you're trying to lose those proverbial 10 pounds to fit into a wedding dress, rock a bathing suit on your next vacation, or surprise everyone at the high school reunion, you have to ask yourself: *What happens once the wedding, vacation or reunion is over?*

In the past, as a newly qualified trainer, I was guilty of using weight loss as the main metric for gauging fitness success. I tried shortcuts, such as calorie-reduced diets, "fat burner" workouts and just about anything else I could to help my clients drop some pounds and reach their weight goal. However, once this was achieved, it was too easy for them to fall right back into old habits. Why? Because I, and my past clients, never thought beyond losing the weight.

> "I have battled with weight issues and an unhealthy lifestyle for what seems like forever. Dai and Christie challenged me, guided me and made me commit to myself. I would still be on my comfy couch if it had not been for them." —JIM

> ## "A man's health can be judged by which he takes two at a time— pills or stairs."
>
> —JOAN WELSH

With this book, I hope to both educate and inspire you to develop a better understanding of fitness, one that's based on how *your* body functions and feels—today, tomorrow and for the rest of your life.

FUN-CTIONAL FITNESS

Let's stop the insanity of a vanity-based approach to fitness, and start prioritizing a function-based understanding of fitness. This, as I like to call it, is *FUN-ctional fitness*, with a big emphasis on the fun. This means taking an enjoyable, exciting and uplifting approach to health and well-being, one that's grounded in real life, not the numbers on a scale, or the size of your pants. Foremost, it's a lifestyle. It's about tying our goals to a lifetime quest to be the best that we can be.

To have a sense of direction on that quest, we need to ask ourselves: *How do I want to feel in 10, 20 or 40 years' time? What quality of life do I want to have now, and when I'm older?*

Be honest with yourself, and you'll start to visualize a new path. You'll start to see how fitness is the very thing that allows you to perform everyday functions, from sitting and getting up, carrying groceries from your car, lifting your child, playing with your grandchild, or putting together a piece of IKEA furniture (don't laugh, that's actually one tough workout!). In these everyday scenarios, we're recruiting the same muscle groups that are used in the conditioning movements I explain in Chapters 7 and 8.

So using that chair (or sitting on the toilet, for that matter) mimics a squat. Lifting your groceries from the floor to the counter, then from the counter to the cupboard, combines a deadlift, bicep curl and shoulder press all in one fluid movement. And simply getting up from a prone position is the basis of a burpee. (What's that? Never heard of a burpee? Turn to page 92 if you can't contain your curiosity!)

We may take these daily actions for granted, but if we don't look after ourselves, or consider our fitness on a daily basis, our muscles and bones will deteriorate with age, and our mobility will be restricted, compromising even the simplest of movements. After all, there's truth to the old adage: *Use it or lose it.* That is, losing the ability to move your body unassisted results in a serious downturn in your quality of life. Think about it: We all know the importance of investing and saving for our future financial security, but what daily investments do we make in our health?

Will a FUN-ctional fitness-focused program improve your appearance? Absolutely. Is that the ultimate end goal? No! FUN-ctional fitness energizes you in every moment of your life. It gives you confidence in the knowledge that you're prepared to tackle—if not conquer—whatever physical or mental challenges that life throws at you. You'll be able to do the things that you enjoy now, and as you age. Just as changing the oil in your car makes it run better, FUN-ctional fitness is all about tuning up your body so it can smoothly carry you through your life.

If you're like most people who build a fitness routine into their everyday life, you'll eventually want to complement it with other activities, like playing sports, hiking and playing with your kids. Can you see how fitness is about much more than how you look?

Beyond the physical, great fitness feeds into all aspects of your life. I've trained many folks who initially get into fitness to lose weight. They are spurred on by little victories as they progress, and of course it's great to see them light up with their improved results. I hear them say things like, "I'm down a dress size," or, "I don't remember the last time I was able to tie up my own shoes."

But that's only the beginning. I know my clients are on the right path when I hear them say, "Wow, I haven't woken up with this kind of energy for 10 years," or, "O-M-G! When I used to bring in the groceries, my back would hurt," or, "I used to get winded just from going upstairs to get my laundry. Now I can do this stuff with ease."

I feel pumped when I see clients put their mental energy toward achieving a particular health and fitness goal, such as when parents come to me, wanting to be a positive role model for their kids. They know they need to be healthy and functionally fit in order to run around the park. They know their kids learn by example. And they choose to show them how to live a healthy, active life that's full of vitality, not vanity.

THE FIVE FS

The Whole Life Fitness Power 30 program incorporates the Five Fs, which I like to think of as a house with four walls supporting a great big roof. The walls are: Fitness, Family, Faith

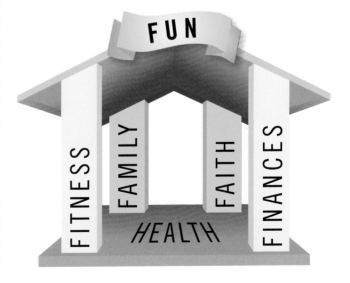

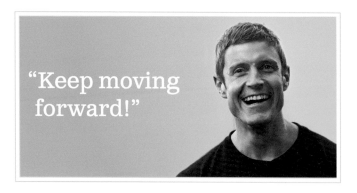

"Keep moving forward!"

and Finances, while the roof that over-arches everything is the fifth F: FUN! The rock-solid foundation of good health and well-being lies beneath everything—and that's what you want to build your "house" upon.

We've already started to explore the first F: fitness. What about the others?

FAMILY

Family, to me, means your tribe of special people, regardless of whether you are related by blood. This may be your partner and children, or your siblings and parents, but it can also include your close friends or work colleagues. It's anybody with whom you have an ongoing and deep relationship that grows over time. Your family includes the folks who encourage you to constantly improve yourself.

For me, family primarily means my wife, Christie, and two daughters, Chardonae and Brielyn. I value their opinions above all others. My family means everything to me; they help me maintain my purpose. They are a big reason why I am so motivated to embody the five Fs as diligently as I do. They give meaning and context to many of the decisions I make and offer me insight and guidance. When faced with a tough decision, I often ask myself what my family would think about it. My moral compass is best directed with one question: *Am I being the type of man I would want my daughters to marry?* If the answer is *no*, then I have to challenge myself with other questions: *Why did I act that way; why did I have that thought; why did I speak that way to my wife?*

Do you see where I'm going with this? If you're still not sure what I mean, let's explore the other side of the coin. What if you didn't have the support of your family, close friends, co-workers and peers? How would that make you feel?

If I were to say to one of my daughters, when they were facing a challenge, "Give up now; you're never going to get it," how would the *family* wall of her house look? I might as well knock it down with a sledgehammer.

I've coached many people who have told me that their family doesn't support them on their path to becoming healthier. For example, "My husband loves me, but he keeps bringing home pizza and chips for the kids, when he knows I want to start eating better," or, "I really feel alone. No one believes I can do it. Heck, *I* don't know if I can do it. Why am I doing this, and what's the point?"

We need connection and a sense of belonging to our group, team, or tribe—our *family*. It's a slippery slope we find ourselves on when we've either lost, or never had, that kind of support. We tend to drift aimlessly through life when we feel isolated and alone. But when you feel happy and loved, flavours take on new dimension, and colours seem more vibrant.

In *Social: Why Our Brains Are Wired to Connect*, neuroscientist Matthew Lieberman explains how the human need to connect is as fundamental to our survival as food and water. Children feel hurt when their social bonds are threatened or cut, which increases the likelihood of health and academic problems later in life.

Personally, I think John Lennon said it best: *All you need is love*.

Of course, we're all human, with complex emotions that sometimes get the best of us. It's only natural to lose our cool from time to time, and to disagree with the people closest to us. I know I've had less-than-proud moments when I have lost my temper with my family. All through the day, all I would think about was how I'd lashed out at my wife or children, replaying the scene in my mind over and over again. I'd feel so badly about myself that I would make bad decisions at work and eat poorly, if at all. Those times really sucked!

THE POWER OF HUMAN CONNECTION

Human connection is an incredibly powerful motivator. In the past, our ancestors valued human touch and close interactions with one another. This need for empathetic touch remains important today. For example, studies have shown that babies in orphanages have higher mortality rates when they aren't cuddled and socially stimulated. Speaking from personal experience, I know that the power of a hug from my kids, a caress from my wife, or even a congratulatory high-five or fist-pump from a friend or colleague puts a huge pep in my step and elevates my motivation.

The seemingly simple action of physical human connection can lift a person from a place of self-doubt to a place of self-belief. I've seen this over and over again with my clients: a gentle pat on the back, helping someone up from the floor after a set of sit-ups—any small act of kindness involving a light touch is enough to make a connection, and BAM!, the other person lights up. Next thing you know, they pay it forward and use that energy to tackle their life with a newfound appreciation, passion, and understanding.

To test this idea, try to recall a time in your life when you felt deflated or depressed. Take a bad day at work, or a time when you lost your temper with your child. Maybe your GPA has been brought down by that C on a final exam; or you gained an extra pound this week, even though you're sure you followed your program perfectly. All of these scenarios suck! Yes, I said suck. It's okay to say that—you can't be positive all of the time. (Seriously, we're only human.) Can you think of the difference it would make, if, in any of those situations, someone you cared about took the time to console you?

I see this in my kids, when they feel down about something. A simple, loving touch on the shoulder, or a few words of encouragement is all it really takes to help them feel happier, more confident, and ready to take on whatever is getting them down.

Empathy is more than a powerful emotion. I believe it's an important life skill, one that everyone should practise. Taking the time to understand each other and our feelings can make a very big difference in the world.

Of course, I'd always apologize when I went home to Christie and my girls. I'd acknowledge that I wasn't the dad or husband I aspired to be, and ask for their forgiveness. And until they felt ready to forgive me, I wasn't myself.

My family bond is the mortar between the bricks and tiles of my house—and I'm their wall, too.

Christie and I now have a rule in our home, and I encourage you to adopt it in yours. Our family mantra is, "Fight fast; make up faster!" We might disagree and even argue once in a while, but we make a point of getting it all out on the table, leaving nothing to chance or second guesses. We strive to get to the understanding and agreement quickly, and move on. This has worked wonders for us, and I know it can help you, too. Just try it and see how it affects the quality of your relationships. If I'm wrong, so be it. (But let's not fight about it... LOL.)

FAITH

For many people, the word *faith* is synonymous with *God* and *religion*, but my definition is much broader. Faith is the underlying principle of believing in something beyond yourself. This could be as simple as a belief in the essential goodness of humankind, or a sense of inter-connectedness with all living things. It's this spirit, this positive driving force and sense of purpose that fuels your courage as well as your optimism in life.

The meaning that we make of our everyday lives is what gives us a sense of direction, which is so crucial to feeling fulfilled. You wouldn't jump into your car and drive without a destination in mind. The same can be said of our lives when we make decisions by default, without giving them much thought. Doesn't it make sense to be more conscious about what we are doing and where we are going?

Surrounding ourselves with quality people is key to my family.

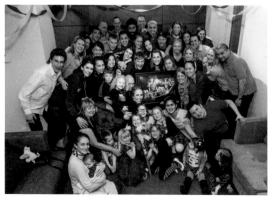

My sense of direction comes from my desire to create positive energy and help people. I have faith that other people feel the same way, wanting to be part of a movement to eliminate, or at least reduce, stress.

I take a leaf out of my daughters' book. Christie and I have raised them to have a positive mindset, which has seemed to help them make new friends quickly. When we take them to the park, they're open and friendly toward the other kids because they expect to find some goodness there. Why can't adults exude this type of positivity more often?

Studies have shown that when we are highly focused on one thing, we often miss out on noticing the unexpected. At times this selectivity prevents us from seeing some of the most wondrous sights right under our noses: the vibrant yellow hues of a daffodil; the fiery reds of a rose bush in bloom; the baby duck in tow behind its mother and siblings; or simply the grass blades bending in the wind. These are all little miracles in and of themselves. What if we could focus on seeing the positive in others and in the world around us? How would that affect our lives?

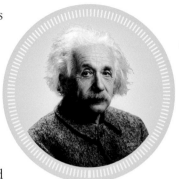

"The measure of intelligence is the ability to change"
—ALBERT EINSTEIN

Take *The Invisible Gorilla*, a book based on the work of researchers Christopher Chabris and Daniel Simons. They found that when people focus so hard on something, they become blind to everything else, including the most unexpected—even when it's right in front of their eyes! This phenomenon is called "intentional blindness," and once developed, it becomes easy for a person to miss out on little details. In truth, I think that many of us fail to take notice of life's amazing landscapes because we are too focused on the ground beneath our feet, or at times, the devices glued to our hands. It's time to lift our heads and take it all in.

FINANCES

Financial stability is a cornerstone of any happy life. Whether you have a little or a lot of money, living within your means gives you security and peace of mind. For most of us, buying the things we want as soon as we want them brings short-term satisfaction, but living above our means puts a lot of strain on our lives. When you're buried under debt, you're carrying a load that relentlessly weighs on you both physically and psychologically. How can anyone relax and be happy when one of the walls of their house is crumbling? It's impossible!

Paying attention to your finances, and being realistic about what you really need to spend money on are two ways to be financially fit.

Ask yourself how you want to live when you reach retirement. Would you like to travel around the world? Spend the summers golfing in Australia and the winters skiing in the Swiss Alps? The range of options available to you will vary based on your financial health in your golden years, but the more financially fit you are now, the more golden those years will be.

Speaking from personal experience, it wasn't until I committed to a "forced savings" model that I started amassing funds. I set up a savings account with automatic monthly transfers, and in 12 years, I was amazed at how much I had put aside.

Of course, I believe that consulting with a financial planner is the best way to go, as I'm a big believer in working with industry experts for assistance in improving the areas of my life where I know I need help. It's beyond my area of expertise, or the scope of this book, to offer anyone financial advice. But, as a personal lifestyle coach, I do ask my clients how they think of their future. That's because you want to increase your ability to live a life full of *YES* opportunities. (By the way, if you are looking for some great resources to help you with your financial fitness, check out the recommended reading list on my blog.)

FUN

Each strong wall contributes to the fun we experience! That's why fun is the roof in the "house" of the five Fs. Ensuring your family, faith, finances and fitness involve fun is key to enjoying your life, and moving through life with a fun-loving attitude is only possible when all of the other elements are strong and healthy.

Fun can be a great motivator to move your body, too. For example, in Stockholm, Sweden, a public staircase was modified to look and sound like a piano. People "played" the "notes" as they climbed or descended the staircase. In this experiment, more than 60 per cent of participants chose to climb the piano rather than take the escalator, just for the fun of it! And in Moscow, during the Sochi Winter Olympics, commuters were given free rides on the subway if they performed 30 squats. So cool.

No matter what your personal priorities or goals, the five Fs are integral to a richer, happier life. Like the walls of a house, the integrity of the whole structure is compromised if any one of the five Fs is weak.

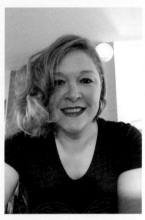

"I stumbled onto Dai Manuel's blog from deep in my couch and got the chance to be a member of the Whole Life Fitness Manifesto community. Sometimes it's hard to find the motivation to do ANYTHING, but Dai pushes, cajoles, and encourages you to take a step, then another, and another. It's never more than you can handle, but he reminds you that there is always room for improvement." —CATHERINE

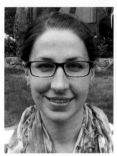

"Unlike other programs that focus on drastic changes in a short amount of time, the Whole Life Fitness Power 30 provides practical and realistic strategies to increase your health, happiness, and gratitude, and they all flow into other aspects of my daily life. When you feel happier, stronger, and more energetic, and when you are mindful of how you nourish your body, you naturally gain a new sense of self-worth, a desire to try new things, and a commitment to make positive changes in all aspects of your life. You spread joy and happiness because it feels good...YOU feel good. And if you have a hard day, you don't feel like you failed, because there are so many ways to be successful in this program." —AMANDA

Taking care of the five Fs is about getting more out of your *whole* life. With a solid platform of underlying health, the body becomes an instrument through which you can achieve everything else. Creating a fitness regime that is focused on daily maintenance instead of vanity-based short-term goals will enable you to have the best possible quality of life as you age, and that changes how you approach everything. This is what I mean by holistic fitness. The mind, body and spirit make up a powerful team. Allow them to support each other, and they will take you far.

IT'S UP TO YOU!

Most importantly, the *Whole Life Fitness Manifesto* is about the choices *you* make, rather than outside forces. As a trainer, I often see habitual externalizing, that is, clients putting the blame on people or situations other than themselves. I hear things like, "I got a flat tire today, so I couldn't show up for my training session with you. Guess I'm not going to be able to work out today." That person encountered an

> "The Whole Life Fitness Power 30 is a well thought-out, easy-to-follow program focused on self-improvement. Every aspect has been covered, from mindfulness to personal development, including helpful links to websites with exercise demonstrations. This program is both thoughtful and practical. As a coach, Dai is incredibly supportive, making himself available for any question or concern you might have; he also reaches out and checks in if he hasn't heard from you in a few days. He is genuine in his commitment and passion for wanting everyone to succeed." —COLLEEN

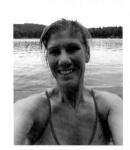

> "As a working mom of three, Dai has really helped me to dedicate what little time I have to my personal growth: mind, body, and spirit. Through the Whole Life Fitness Power 30, I am stronger, healthier, and smaller (I've lost a total of 12 pounds and two dress sizes). People in my life have been commenting on my physical abilities, appearance, and dedication to my health; now I'm the one inspiring others! I have completed a leg of a triathlon, Tough Mudder, and I recently signed up for another obstacle race." —CAREY

external force that disrupted their schedule, and they allowed it to disrupt their commitment to themselves. They decided it was okay not to follow through because they have a convenient cop-out. The truth is, in most situations the externalization just boils down to an internal dialogue. *You've* made a choice. You've chosen to allow that to be the reason why you can't follow through on the commitment you made. Of course, life is unpredictable and sometimes stuff happens, but usually, it's really just a matter of setting priorities.

Being a working parent of two girls, I acutely understand the pressures of a challenging schedule. My daughters need to be driven to extra-curricular activities or birthday parties, and suddenly there's an extra squeeze on the time I put aside for exercise. When this happens, I know that I simply *have* to find time later or earlier in the day, but my commitment must remain in place. I'm careful to avoid leaning on the *no-time* crutch, along with other all-too-common excuses. There really is truth to the expression: *Excuses are just bad habits in disguise.*

I often stay motivated by remembering people who I find inspiring, and this trick might help you, too. If you consider what today's highest achievers have in common, you'll find that mental rigour plays a big role in their successes. Prime examples include Oprah Winfrey, global entrepreneur Richard Branson, author and business coach Marie Forleo, motivational speaker Robin Sharma, leadership expert Simon Sinek and scholar Brené Brown. All of these people have a no-quit attitude; they believe, and they follow-through.

In particular, I see life success coach Anthony Robbins as someone who embodies this principle. Robbins aims to inspire people to take control of their lives, to fulfil their potential and be the best that they can be. He also leads by example. Take, for instance, Robbins's philosophy of gratitude. While teaching the importance of gratitude, Robbins happens to be one of the most globally influential philanthropists, giving both his time and money to the causes that are important to him.

Author Simon Sinek has made it his life's mission to inspire leaders and help people realize their underlying driving purpose. In *Start With Why: How Great Leaders Inspire Everyone to Take Action*, Sinek encourages readers to identify their purpose, and create a life geared toward fulfilling it. When you have that drive and your spirit is on fire, you wake up in the morning with a hop, skip and a jump. Do you think a person in that mental state wants to go and exercise? Heck, yeah, because they are in the right frame of mind to have fun while they do it! They're already energized so they are naturally drawn to activities that will energize them even more. Our bodies instinctively know that one of the best ways to keep that energy high is simply to elevate our heart rate on a regular basis.

The language you use is crucial to connecting your goals to your ability to achieve them. Replace *I can't* with *I can*, and you will find that it leads to *I do; I will*. Replace *discipline* with *desire*, and you may find that you feel less bullied by your internal monologue, and more motivated. Guilt and blame have no place in the *Whole Life Fitness Manifesto*.

And this is where physical and mental fitness really start to reinforce each other in a positive feedback loop. We all know we need to push past physical resistance when we're working out, on a strenuous hike, or skiing or snowboarding down a tough mountain run. It's mental focus that comes to our rescue and carries us forward when our muscles start to fatigue. We need healthy thoughts and loving self-talk to encourage ourselves to take care of our bodies, and to face the challenges that life throws at us. In turn, a strong, healthy body will give you the energy, confidence and the sense of bounce you need to achieve your goals.

Of course, there's nothing wrong with bringing in reinforcements, especially when you're just starting out. I'll sometimes joke with my clients, "There's nothing more

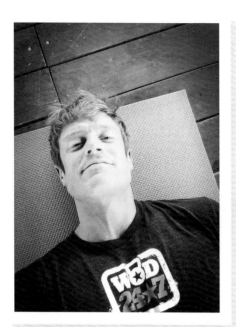

I think I got savasana figured out, does that make me a yogi?

motivating than my size 12 shoe connecting with your butt." Kidding aside, I do understand how a trainer can be motivating, especially at the beginning of a new fitness regime. Accountability is a great motivator, and that added sense of camaraderie, or community, makes working out a lot more fun!

THE IMPORTANCE OF MINDFULNESS

Mindfulness is a bit of a buzzword these days, and for good reason. To me, it is simply a feeling of mental clarity. It means cultivating awareness, not only of my body but also of my place in the world. We're reactionary creatures by nature, and that tendency is compounded by so many stimuli being fired at us at all times, especially from media and the advertising industry.

In an interview with CBS, advertising executive Jay Walker-Smith said that we're exposed to up to 5,000 ad messages a day, which is a steep hike from the 500 or so we saw daily in the 1970s. While this may seem impossibly high, the truth is we are hit with brand impressions from the moment we wake up until we go to bed, thanks in large part to the prevalence of the Internet in our daily lives. Just think of the number of brand messages that bombard you, just on your smartphone alone. Every day, the massive amount of media messages we receive is a huge drain on our mental energy.

I find that my best time for really connecting with where I'm at is right after a hard workout. I'm physically taxed, lying on my back on the ground stretching out into what the yogis call *savasana*, or the corpse pose. I lie with my eyes closed, feet and knees gently falling open, shoulders relaxed and my arms by my side with the palms facing upwards. My breathing becomes shallower as my mind focuses on the job of relaxation. As each thought comes to me, I acknowledge it before gently pushing it away. It's in this state that I can really tune into my body and reach a higher state of mental clarity.

Of course there are many other forms of mindfulness practice and meditation (which we'll get into in Chapter 5), but I love *savasana* because it's simple and works for everyone. Just taking that five, 10 or 15 minutes to be still inevitably calms the mind, so that your ideas can flow. In fact, many of my most creative ideas come to me after *savasana*, such as a conversation that I need to have, or a new project that I want to start. For me, that's where that mind-body connection happens, and it packs a powerful punch.

During *savasana*, I start to feel like I am just being; I don't feel pressure to make decisions, because I am able to simply be present and in the moment. I'm not worried about past decisions; I'm not concerned about what tomorrow will bring—I'm simply cognizant of my existence in that moment of stillness. I'm there with breathing, and my gratitude for being there. That's the idea behind the *Whole Life Fitness Manifesto*, to bring you into this state of ease and alignment, where everything's just trucking along, feeling good.

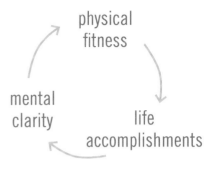

And here's the kicker: It's all a positive upward spiral! After incorporating these practices into your life for a while—body and mind both healthy and feeling good—you'll start to experience a deeply satisfying cycle of mental clarity, physical fitness and life accomplishments, where everything feeds each other.

Our minds are a culmination of everything that's happened before now. For me, that includes every action I've taken, every food I've eaten, and every person I've met. Is it possible to get physically fit without taking care of your mental and spiritual self? Sure. But it's harder to get going, and it's less fun along the way.

THE WHOLE LIFE FITNESS POWER 30

I designed the Whole Life Fitness Power 30 in such a way that you don't have to reinvent your lifestyle to accommodate it. Instead, you can plug this 30-minute ritual into your busy day. Each 30-minute session breaks down like this:

1. 15 minutes for your workout of the day (WOD), or movement with purpose
2. 5 minutes for meditation or mindfulness
3. 10 minutes of concentrated personal development

Think about this: 30 minutes makes up just two per cent of your 24-hour day. This time is just for you—no excuses. Commit to it the same way you commit to brushing your teeth, and I promise you'll see big shifts in your whole life.

Remember, you're not alone on this journey—I'm here for you; I'll show you the way, both in this book and in our online community. So let's get into a huddle and start making some awesome changes in our lives—together!

UNLIMITED
POSSIBILITIES

Creative
projects

INDEPENDENCE

Feel
free
to do
whatever
moves
me

Have a healthy l♥ve life

WHAT'S THE REASON WHY YOU WANT **WHOLE LIFE FITNESS?**

Be a
GREAT
parent

Don't BUY
happiness
— BE
happiness

SELF-RESPECT

JOY 😊 LOVE

Travel the world

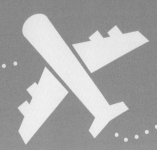

DISCOVER YOUR PERSONAL *WHY*

CHAPTER 2

SO WHY DO WE—OR SHOULD we—care about all of this, anyway? What's the point of getting fit or sharpening our mind?

Well, let's reverse those questions for a minute. Put simply, what's the point of *not* being healthy and fit? Of *not* being mentally sharp? Why would any of us *not* want to fulfil our potential?

I believe that the five Fs—Fitness, Family, Faith, Finances and FUN—are the cornerstones of happiness. And of course we all want to be happy! The trouble crops up when we focus on short-term goals rather than thinking about life as a whole. We get lost in dealing with our day-to-day schedules, chasing immediate gratification, or just reacting to whatever life is throwing at us in any given moment. But once you start to widen your focus to your whole life, those walls and roof all start to matter a lot more.

If you have kids in your life, watching them grow up can be a powerful reminder of how fast time ticks by. When we're just dealing with our own lives day in, day out, we don't notice the passage of time so much, but there's nothing like the wonderful wake-up call of witnessing your children develop new skills and learn new things. Who wants to look back five years down the road and suddenly say, "Hey, what the heck did I do with that half decade of my life?"

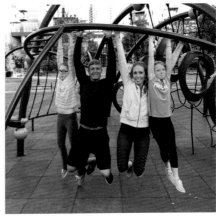

I plan to be fit to play at any age.

Having a passion, or a deep-rooted sense of purpose, helps to guide the choices you make. Even big decisions become much easier to navigate, eventually becoming more consistent with the plan you have for your life overall. Time still passes, of course, but you won't suddenly wonder where it all went.

Of course, you have to have flexibility and be prepared to adjust your plan from time to time. Things change along the path of any journey, and we all have to re-route when we run up against roadblocks (or speed bumps, as I prefer to think of them). But even course-correction is much easier to deal with when we're in line with our purpose, passion, or beliefs, and when we have a clear sense of our direction.

In the end, it's about being intentional about what you want to get out of your life. What are the experiences you're creating for yourself right NOW that will become the stories you'll tell later? Will they be stories you're proud of? If your life experiences are ones that you're truly happy to shout about, and can look back on with pride and satisfaction, they add up to a life well lived.

MY WHY

My personal *why* is all about connecting with people, whether it is my family, my friends, or my tribe. This drive for connection to others underscores my very being. It's a vital, addictive source of enjoyment in my life. I get a huge kick out of being able to help others become healthier and happier; this gives me my *joie de vivre* that makes me jump out of bed every morning. The more people I reach, the greater the impact on my online community, as other leaders invariably emerge to carry forward this fitness movement, like ripples on a pond.

For the past several years, my whole family has come to the gym with me bright and early on Sunday mornings to teach an awesome group of people keen to learn the *Whole Life Fitness Manifesto* way of being. Hundreds of people have attended these *Sunday Funday* events, helping me to realize my goal of improving the lives of as many people as possible. These weekly events are like little beacons of light that remind me of my purpose.

My personal *why* can be boiled down to: *I'm here to help people live happy, healthier, more active lifestyles while developing richer, deeper and more meaningful personal relationships with themselves, and their friends, families, and communities.*

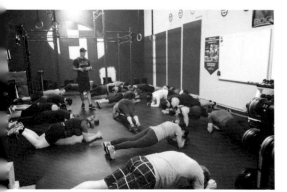

Leading our Sunday Funday tribe is a big part of fulfilling my personal *why.*

HOW IT ALL STARTED

My own personal *why* is deeply rooted in my past as a morbidly obese teenager.

When I was nine, my parents announced they were divorcing and it rocked my world. Until that moment, I had thought I had the perfect life, so I struggled hard with this traumatic event. Suddenly, all I wanted was to *be wanted*. At that time, only one other child at my school had separated parents, which added extra social stigma to my experience.

I withdrew from friends, family, social outings—life experiences—and tried to fill the void I felt within, which mainly involved eating. Our family dinners were well-rounded, but outside of mealtimes, I was a junk-food junkie. Food was my crutch. Very quickly, I developed a bad habit of reaching for more snacks than I should, choosing burgers, fries and other garbage that barely landed in my stomach before I wanted more. In hindsight, I can see that I was making choices without really understanding why I made them. I was on autopilot, just acting on an impulse to soothe my turbulent emotions.

I certainly didn't offload those extra calories with anything even approaching an active lifestyle. Blame it on too much time playing video games, too much lounging in front of the TV, combined with a lack of education around where my sedentary lifestyle was heading.

By the time I reached puberty, my frame—then 167 cm (5 ft 6 in) in height—weighed in at about 90 kg (200 lbs), with a 96-cm (38-in) waist.

The usual emotional and physical upheavals of adolescence made the situation even worse. As anyone who is or has been overweight knows, there's a stigma that comes with being large. People can be cruel, but teenagers downright vicious in their ridicule. My peers found it hard to even look me in the eye and I was well aware of their snickering—behind my back, and even right in my face. I understood; I avoided looking at my own body when I stepped out of the shower. I wore baggy clothing in an attempt to camouflage my protruding belly. And shorts? I never wore them, no matter how hot the weather might be.

I said *no* to everything. Attend a pool party where I would have to wear a bathing suit? *No way!* Participate in gym class? *Out of the question.* Go to a school dance? *No thanks.* I'd simply avoid anything physical, leveraging my asthma as an excuse to opt out.

Through these lifestyle choices, I soon became freighted with low self-esteem. I approached rock bottom, feeling depressed and isolated. I can admit now that I even had suicidal thoughts.

And then one Sunday morning, I decided to do something that I usually avoided: I looked at my reflection in the mirror. Up to that point, I was able to pretend that things weren't as bad as they were, because I wasn't looking the problem in the eye. *Deny, deny, deny.* Facing up, however, I broke down in tears. I had never felt so low

HOW ACTIVE ARE OUR KIDS?

Physical inactivity is now identified as the 4th leading risk factor for global mortality. The WHO Physical Activity Guidelines recommend that kids from 5 to 17 years old should get at least 60 minutes of moderate to vigorous intensity physical activity every day. What's unfortunate is that many children in first world countries aren't achieving this minimum.

SOURCE: WORLD HEALTH ORGANIZATION

in my life. At that moment, I experienced an epiphany: I really didn't like where my life was going.

I knew that deep down, I enjoyed life. At least, I had enjoyed it before, and I wanted to enjoy it again. I faced a simple choice: to remain this way forever, or to do something about it. So I picked myself up and deliberately shifted my *poor me* attitude. In that moment, I recalibrated my motivation. I reasoned my way to a decision. And then I made a change.

I hit the library and pored over books on health, nutrition and fitness. (Yes, I did all of this pre-Google!) I started eating a little less and moving a little more. I started slowly with walking daily, then mountain biking. I strapped on my cassette player (yes I'm dating myself here), with a tape playing on endless loop (A side to B side to A and so on), I'd ride until I had exhausted both the tape and myself. Only then would I would ride home.

I added more and more daily activity incrementally, eventually joining a gym. Over 14 months, I was transformed. This time, adolescence itself was on my side as I shot up to over 185 cm (6 ft 1 in)—a growth spurt that doubtlessly helped to burn some calories! My weight didn't change that much, but I saw body fat melt away as new lean muscle mass appeared. Now, with a better understanding of the science and biology of health, I know that my physical changes came from a combination of cardiovascular and resistance training. I strengthened my body, increasing my lean muscle, which cranked up my metabolism (my body's natural furnace). I felt stronger, healthier and

I understand what it's like to struggle with excess weight because I've been there myself.

more confident in my abilities to tackle whatever physical obstacles stood in my way. Rather than saying *no* to pool parties and gym class, I started asking people to join *me* in activities. I felt good. I was alive.

I've never gone back to that state of obesity, but I don't forget what it was like. This helps me to relate to my clients who face weight challenges. I know how it feels when people stare at you. I know what it's like to be out of breath from climbing a flight of stairs, or to have difficulty with something as simple as tying your shoes. When you're struggling physically, sometimes it's the little things that seem the hardest to do. If this describes you right now, I want you to know that you're not alone, and that it doesn't have to stay this way.

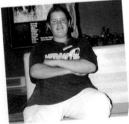

Dai Manuel - 14 yrs old

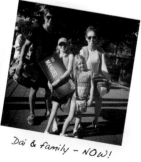

Dai & family - NOW!

In the years that followed, everything seemed to go in the right direction. In 2001, I met my life partner, Christie, and we had two wonderful daughters. I achieved success in my business life as Chief Operating Officer and founding partner of Fitness Town, a chain of fitness equipment stores. I also became a Level 1 Coach of the popular strength and conditioning program, CrossFit.

But I reached a pivotal point at age 32, when, despite having a wonderful family, strong physical fitness and some professional success, I felt untethered. I had become obsessed with physical fitness, and while that meant I had achieved my goal weight, I hadn't done anything to heal myself emotionally and spiritually. There were underlying issues that I hadn't dealt with, so I strayed from the very things that should have brought me the most happiness.

If I look at my life in terms of the five Fs, I can easily see why my house was crumbling at the time. I was physically and financially fit, but I wasn't paying enough attention to the state of my faith or my family. I was a fractured person on a downward spiral, having little fun, and this cast a shadow over my entire life. I was depressed and disconnected, and felt like I was headed for a midlife crisis—and I wasn't anywhere near midlife!

Even though I had lost all that extra weight as a teenager, I was still burdened by shame and guilt. I still saw myself as unattractive and unlovable. So when I started becoming successful, I binged on other people's attention. I craved validation from others, because I had felt deprived of approval for so long. I neglected and disrespected both my family and myself.

It was Christie who brought me back to what was important to me. I saw that I didn't really need approval from the whole world, and that that kind of attention would never satisfy me anyway. What I really needed was a steady and secure connection with the people most important to me: my wife and daughters.

Christie has always seen something in me that I couldn't see in myself then. She saw me as the man that I *wanted* to be, and helped me choose to be that person. Similar to the epiphany I experienced when I was 15, I realized that I was the only person who could really turn my life around.

> "It all starts with clarity. You have to know WHY you do WHAT you do."
>
> —*START WITH WHY*
> AUTHOR SIMON SINEK

I started by taking inventory of my life at that moment. Now let me just say, this is not an easy task for anyone. It takes brutal honesty and a willingness to explore past choices and paths travelled. Whether the outcomes were good or bad, this exercise is not meant to create stress, anxiety, guilt or regret. It's simply an exercise to recreate the road map of our life, in order to understand what has brought us to where we are today. Through understanding our path, we can gain valuable insights to help us better navigate or change our course.

When I underwent this exercise of introspection, I felt much like Dorothy exposing the Wizard of Oz behind that proverbial curtain. I had erected many façades to portray myself as what I believed to be a "success." I worked long, hard hours as I chased a professional title and recognition, but often at the cost of my family and friends. My physical and mental health suffered with the added pressure of the expectations I had set for myself. With no outlet for my mounting stress, I continued to withdraw and immerse myself in my work, thinking that would make me feel better. I was wrong. Admittedly, I was very proud of my work ethic, which I had learned from my parents. But without stability and balance in my personal life, the walls of my house bowed like blades of grass in the wind. Something had to change.

In retrospect, I don't look at my decision to pursue my career as a mistake, but as an opportunity to learn what is most important to me. At that moment, I made a decision to put my family and personal health ahead of my career. Over time, as I committed to daily physical exercise, I found that my health improved and my stress decreased. I spent focused time with my wife and daughters every single day—no matter what else I was doing, they came first. And do you know what happened? My career advanced. I found I was even *more* productive at work because I knew that I had to maximize my time on the job. My mindset had shifted a full 180 degrees, and I now cherished time with family and friends, along with my daily ritual of physical exercise.

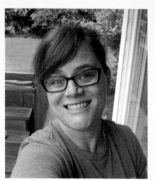

"Dai and his Whole Life Fitness Power 30 have helped me get through one of the most difficult times of my adult life. Even when I wasn't following the program, his voice was in my head, telling me that I could get through this. The lessons I've learned from him have helped me to go forward, with confidence in myself." —ERIN

One of the first things I did to get back on the positivity train was giving up alcohol. I had started to use booze to calm myself; it was my numbing agent.

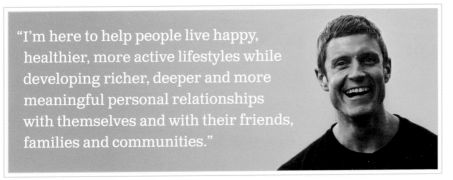

"I'm here to help people live happy, healthier, more active lifestyles while developing richer, deeper and more meaningful personal relationships with themselves and with their friends, families and communities."

When I felt the responsibilities of life bearing down on me, it was easier to uncork a bottle of wine or crack a beer than it was to deal with things head on.

I knew that my habit of reaching for the bottle was connected to my feelings of unhappiness. Since I was actively trying to create more happiness in my life, I had to make a choice. I made my decision, and made it known to my family, friends and co-workers. It was a very challenging transition, but an awesome one that I will forever be glad I made. Of course, it can be tough to deal with life's stresses at times—that never goes away—but knowing that I feel those stresses for everything that they are is far better than feeling numb.

FINDING FAITH

The process of healing really began when I uncovered my own personal faith. Maybe it's because I majored in philosophy at university; I tend to ponder over the same questions, such as: *Why am I here?*, *What's my life all about?*, *What can I do to make the world a better place?*, and finally, *Is this all there is?*

I realized that the things I wanted to gain in life didn't match my daily habits. I was saying one thing and doing something completely different, and to make matters worse, I was bitter at the world for not giving me more. No matter how much success I gained, I never felt satisfied. It was like having an appetite you can never satiate, something that's both debilitating and demotivating.

I knew that I wanted to focus on my personal relationships, as well as my relationship with myself. Additionally, I took control of my own mental inputs, or the information I received through books, TV, social media and other mediums. I could choose the types of messages I wanted in my mind. I began deliberately filling my head with positive messages, books, popular TED Talks and the teachings of influential world leaders, such as Nelson Mandela, Abraham Lincoln and Mahatma Gandhi, to name just a few.

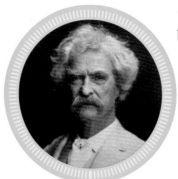

"The two most important days in your life are the day you are born, and the day you find out why."

—MARK TWAIN

And you know what happened? I became more aware and appreciative of the people that made up my communities, both online and offline. I soon saw that I needed to share what I had learned, and to give back to those I wanted to help, and most importantly, those who *wanted* help.

And that was it! At that time, with the positive influence of my wife, I made a conscious decision to put others first. Soon after, my external voice began to sound more like the one in my head. Many amazing things started happening in my life and the lives of those around me.

My faith is not set in a religion per se, but it is founded on a sense that there's something in each of us that wants to give. If we acknowledge that we are lucky to live in a country where we have freedom, and where we can lead a life of our own design, and offer a hand to our fellow human beings, we can make this world an even more amazing place.

My *why* is my purpose, and it provides a filter through which I can weigh my daily choices, actions and responses. My faith lights me up from within, and gives me intention for how I want to live my life. Whether I'm writing a blog entry, posting an update to social media, calling a client, coaching a Sunday Funday class, serving a customer, or helping my family, I do it with 120 per cent enthusiasm and pure, genuine excitement. And I believe that the exercise of self-discovery of your own personal purpose can bring you *your* why, along with infinite joy and satisfaction.

FINDING YOUR WHY

Finding your own *why* is the most important factor to achieving long-term whole life fitness, and it's important to remember that that's going to look different for everyone. Everybody needs to explore their own particular reasons for becoming fit, and make the decision to follow through. It all boils down to feeling (as well as fuelling) the desire to make a change, and then doing it.

So, what do you need to ask yourself? There's a reason why you started looking for answers, whether in this book or elsewhere. Respect that impulse. Perhaps it's centred on your physical health and vitality, and that's great! At the same time, examine whether there's another issue in your life that you want to make better, be it a situation in your family, your finances or your faith.

WHAT MOTIVATES US FOR LIFE?

Think about why fitness matters to you. Your primary motivation might be appearance, or it may seem that way at first. Do you want to return to the weight you were ten years ago? Do you want to "look good" in a bikini? People have a remarkable number of *whys* when they start a fitness program.

These goals relate to superficial, top-layer desire, but once you start to peel that back and dig in, you'll find that there's a lot more going on. I'm not saying we should reject the desire to look good; just that when we look beneath that layer of motivation, we will always find something deeper.

When I survey the people I have coached, I find that what drives most is the desire to create a more fulfilling life. If they're considerably overweight, and their clothes don't fit, they don't feel confident in themselves. When they feel winded by going up a flight of stairs, they're not having fun. Mentally, they're exhausted all of the time, and they want it to stop. For others, such as those who have suffered heart attacks or who have life-threatening illnesses, such as diabetes, the *why* might be a basic desire to live.

For some of us, that deeper motivation stems from a desire to support a healthy relationship with our romantic partner. Christie and I are strong believers in the saying: *Couples who sweat together stay together.*

In my work, I've met a lot of accomplished business executives in their 40s, many who were once football or hockey players, but who are now 23 kg (50 lbs) overweight. Their daily choices over the past decade have taken them a long way from their original lifestyle, usually to a detriment of their fitness. Luckily for them, they often remember how good it felt to be strong and to move freely, without discomfort or pain, so they have both an existing appreciation and a compelling argument for what fitness can provide. Naturally, they want to tap back into that sensation of personal health. For these clients, the sheer pleasure of being active is the *why*.

Maybe your goal is to achieve better cardiovascular fitness so you can have an active retirement. The reality for many of us is that we can't travel as much as we'd like while we're in our

Couples who sweat together stay together.

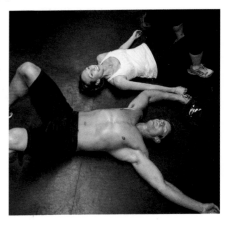

prime and midlife years. We work full-time, we have families to provide for, and older parents who need our time and energy. If you want to be able to see the world when you retire, you'll need to be fit and healthy when you reach that age. Whether your idea of a great travel experience is rising early to watch lions roam freely while on safari in Africa, or stripping down to your swimsuit to wallow in warm Caribbean waters, you'll get more out of it if your body is in an optimal state of health.

Aiming to achieve optimal health is an undoubtedly solid reason to exercise. Now, I know that people have different ideas of what *optimal health* means. For me, health

EXERCISE: THE GOOD, BAD, AND UGLY!

The Good

1. **INCREASED ENERGY**
   You can expect a huge rise in your overall energy on a daily basis.

2. **ENHANCED DEXTERITY**
   You will find your strength and physical coordination improve—navigate the busiest crowds like the ninja you are!

3. **REGULATED APPETITE**
   You might actually feel less hungry, or start to prefer healthy foods that help you fuel the machine.

4. **IMPROVED SLEEP**
   Increased levels of feel-good hormones, such as serotonin, will help you relax more easily at the end of the day and get a proper night's rest.

5. **IMPROVED MOOD**
   If you've ever experienced the "runner's high" then you know how great you can feel at the end of a workout.

6. **GREATER SELF-ESTEEM**
   Self-esteem and confidence stem not just from looking better. You will experience pride as you set fitness goals and reach them.

The Bad

7. **PEER PRESSURE**
   One downside of adopting a healthy lifestyle is you will have to learn to say no on a regular basis. Party invitations and co-workers' birthdays can often derail even the most determined of fitness fiends. Try alternatives— like being the group of friends who crunch rather than lunch together.

8. **INCREASED APPETITE**
   While some people report a decreased appetite, others find that lifting weights and doing more cardio work can make them feel hungrier, as a result of burning up more calories. That's fine, as long as you're eating healthy (see our good nutrition guide in Chapter 6).

9. **BUDGETING**
   Unfortunately, we live in an age of highly processed convenience foods, while their healthier counterparts are often more expensive. Be sure to look out for specials on meats and clearance discounts on fresh produce; this should help your grocery budget stretch a little further.

...and the Ugly!

10. **FREQUENT WASHROOM TRIPS**
    No truly honest exercise article would be complete without mentioning this dirty little secret of fitness enthusiasts. When you're drinking more water, you're likely to need more trips to the washroom.

is about feeling good, being able to function and move about freely, to play with my kids, and feeling able to try a new sport or activity without worrying that I'll injure myself. I like the idea of being able to say *yes* to anything physical, knowing that I'm not limited by my state of health or fitness.

If you're really struggling to find your *why*, try to embrace the process of discovery. Start by analysing your current fitness habits and your general approach to your health. Where can you make a small but sustainable shift? How much water are you drinking per day? Are you getting enough sleep at night? How much time do you spend moving your body each day? Do you exercise at all? Do you play any sports? What do you typically eat? It's all about making little, everyday choices that will improve your health.

If you're feeling beaten down by your current lifestyle, start to feed your brain with positive messages, wherever you find them. It's amazing how often someone else's idea, passion or vision can trigger a feeling or impulse inside *you*. If you're inspired by an event or activity that you read or hear about, go try it! You might surprise yourself, finding that what was once unfamiliar and difficult becomes something that you really love! Start walking a little. It doesn't have to be very much, just something. Get off the couch, walk around the block. Do it today, not tomorrow!

I know that when it comes to health and fitness, it can be scary to try something new. I've seen many people become so used to being overweight or out of shape that they can't imagine any other way of being. Some folks have lived longer in an unhealthy state than they ever did in a healthy one, so they forget what it's like to feel good. But you have to remember: Just because this is how it is now, doesn't mean it has to stay this way. Change is possible. In fact, when you connect with your *why* and commit to following through, I can promise you that change is inevitable.

This applies to all your goals, not just around physical fitness. Whatever is spurring you on, dream big! When I talk to new clients, I always ask them two questions:

1. What do you want to do?
2. Is that all?

Remember that seemingly **HARMLESS CHOICES CAN HAVE A NEGATIVE IMPACT**. Just think of your morning coffee. One teaspoon of sugar and cream represents about 75 calories; in the course of a year, you're looking at an additional 27,375 calories. That's the equivalent of 8 pounds of body weight! And one daily glass of wine—around 150 empty calories—translates to anywhere between 8 to 14 pounds of weight.

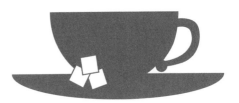

WHAT'S YOUR WHY?

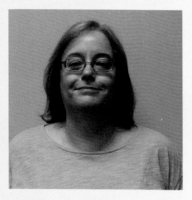

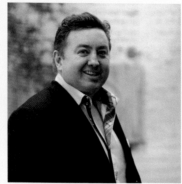

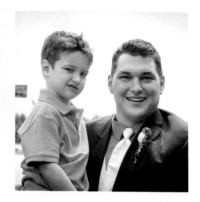

"I want to work on eliminating negative self-talk when I approach, or am in the midst of, any physical challenge. I find it particularly evident in cardio workouts as this is an area of development for me." —KRIS

"I bought a really nice Ted Baker suit, overcoat, and some really nice shirts last year that I cannot wear now. I want to wear them again. I have a number of speaking engagements in Europe and I want to look great. I put on 20 pounds since I bought them (and they were a little tight then) and have lost 10 in the last 6 weeks. I don't want to focus on my weight but rather my shape." —TONY

"I want to be under 245 pounds and run a mile in 8:30. After that I will continue to be healthier with a long-term goal of being 220 pounds at the end of the year and running 1 mile in 7 minutes and 3 miles in 22 minutes. And of course I want to gain muscle because, well, I'm a guy!" —DAVID

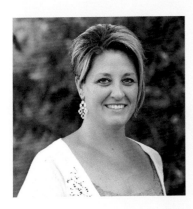

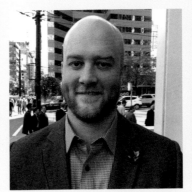

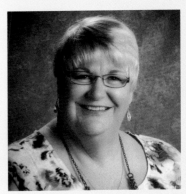

"I'm working towards reducing stress by slowing down, taking things off my schedule, stepping down from some of my responsibilities at work, and delegating more from my to do list. As I subtract things from my life, I'd like to incorporate exercise into my routine and shift my focus to self-care, and start to see this excess weight come off my body."
—MICHELLE

"It seems I have many aches and pains, and not a lot of vitality. I hope to see a huge change in the way my body feels, how I look, and I hope to use this program as a springboard into a regular routine of wellness. I also want to feel good about taking my shirt off (superficial I know, but definitely a mental trigger that would tell me I am doing it). At the end of the day, I want to be healthy to live a long, engaged and active life with my wife and two boys."
—GEOFF

"I want to be 25 pounds lighter and be able to move freely. Using my stairs as a workout, I want to be able to go up and down without stopping for 20 minutes of rest. Right now I can only do one "lap." —JUDI

We #JustDidIt! Conquered our first mud race together, leading a team of 40 courageous individuals. Go team! #IWantMyMudder.

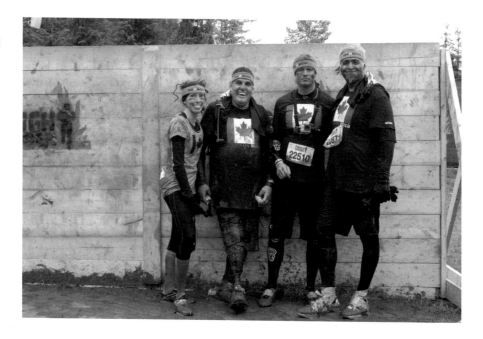

The second question is meant as a challenge, of course. That's because I don't believe in settling for too small a vision of how a good life looks. We are all taught to have impoverished dreams for ourselves and to think that buying things will make us happy. I flip this on its head and say shoot for greatness. That is, *be*—don't buy—happiness.

Just remember: You are not alone. Sometimes success requires us to be humble enough to know that we can't do it all by ourselves, and to reach out to others for help. This is true for everyone; so don't be afraid to ask! Now, I know many people (mainly men) who like to rely on digital shortcuts (Google Maps, anyone?) rather than ask people for help. But you know the most amazing part about turning to each other? Most of us actually want to help! In our super independent society, it's easy to forget that as human beings, we are programmed to care.

HOW FINDING YOUR *WHY* HELPS YOU

As you start to feel better about yourself, life will turn a happy corner. Perhaps you'll enjoy supercharged energy levels. Maybe you will handle stress better, or notice your metabolism working faster. Your life will be filled with good vibes and move along with a sense of bounce. You will think more about health and wellness, and naturally make better food choices. As your energy improves, it's going to be easier to attain all your goals because you will have the drive and power to push yourself. You'll know that feeling better is going to free up so much mental energy and give you the capacity to enjoy all aspects of your life.

So, what's going to fill your bucket? Once you have an idea, then it's a matter of constantly making choices that keep it nice and full.

Let's discover a call to action. Let's all start igniting a sense of discovery in each other. Connecting with your *why* is what will really drive you forward and give you the natural motivation to stay focused on your goal. You made the decision to pick up the *Whole Life Fitness Manifesto*; now you face the decision to put it into action.

> " So, what's going to fill your bucket? Once you have an idea, then it's a matter of constantly making choices that keep it nice and full."

Take **responsibility** instead of **making excuses**

What do *you need* to release in order to do what *you want* to do?

It's a **mental shift**

Who are you making these choices for?

Help yourself first to help others better

GIVE YOUR EXCUSES THE **BOOT**

SPOILER ALERT: Fit people aren't *born* fit; they *work* at it!

Excuses are exactly that: **excuses!**

THERE ARE NO ROADBLOCKS

ONLY SPEED BUMPS

I'M EXHAUSTED AFTER MY COMMUTE–I CAN'T POSSIBLY WORK OUT. ONCE I'VE PUT THE KIDS IN BED, I'M CAN'T AFFORD A GYM MEMBERSHIP. I SPEND TIME DRIVING MY KIDS TO THE SPORTS EXTRA-CURRICULAR ACTIVITIES.

ELIMINATE YOUR
WHY NOTS
CHAPTER 3

MOST PEOPLE HAVE HAD THE experience of starting a new fitness plan, only to abandon it completely or revert back to their old habits. Name one person who hasn't made working out part of their New Year's resolutions at some point in their lives!

We often start with tons of enthusiasm, launching head-on into a brutal workout routine. Perhaps we've tried to cram as much exercise into our downtime as we possibly can, or suddenly begun moving at a pace that's frankly beyond us. Too often the end result is that we crumble as soon as we start feeling even slightly overwhelmed.

It's actually quite possible to become overwhelmed at the very thought of starting to exercise, even before you take the first step. To go from feeling that you don't have the energy to start moving, even a little, to hitting the gym or working with a personal trainer is a huge shift!

Lacking follow-through on a decision to get fit, whether we've started and stopped, or never started at all, usually boils down to a matter of time, fear, energy or motivation.

Who hasn't thought, *I'm too exhausted after my commute to work out*, or, *Once I've put the kids into bed, I'm beat*, or, *I can't work out because I can't afford a gym membership*?

Heck, in my line of work, I've heard it all, including the excuse of, *I'll go to the gym when I'm in better shape.* (Spoiler alert: Fit people aren't born fit; they work at it!) If you use that as your primary excuse, you're *never* going to be fit.

How about this classic line? *I spend all my time driving my kids to their sports and extra-curriculars; it really leaves me with no time left to exercise.* The message you're giving your children is that you're out of shape because of them. And the underlying message is that physical activity is something you have to give up when you become an adult or a parent.

> " I followed Dai for almost two years on social media before attending my first community workout. This man changed my life. He showed me that being busy raising my daughter cannot be an excuse for not exercising but rather it must be the REASON that I do." —MAT

Some people are intimidated—even scared—by the thought of a fitness program, and they simply don't know where to start. They don't know how much time they need to put into it, so they feel unable to create a plan. Others are recovering from an injury, such as a broken leg, in which case remaining inactive might seem like a way to avoid pain or re-injury.

The fact is all of these excuses are exactly that; they are crutches and they stand in the way of our lives. We can choose to allow excuses to prevent us from looking after ourselves. We can use every out at our disposal. Or we can choose to change our mindset.

KICK AWAY THOSE CRUTCHES!

So just how do you kick those metaphorical crutches to the side and stand happily on your own feet? How do you remove your own perceived barriers and flow into that moment when you just *know* what needs to be done, and you're ready to do it? For some people, the best first step toward becoming active is one that may seem paradoxically *inactive*: meditation. I often recommend that my clients ease into The Whole Life Fitness Power 30 by starting with just 15 minutes of mindfulness, and 15 minutes of personal development (there will be more in later chapters on how to spend that time).

This advice may come as a surprise, but I have found that dialling into your mind and spirit is a great place to start, because it offers a solid route to understanding the body's purpose as the vehicle that takes you through life. Taking this type of holistic approach—looking at the mind as well as the body—really helps you to connect with your *why*. This prompts a mental shift into taking responsibility and acting decisively, instead of making excuses. It's important that you avoid pointing the finger or offloading your excuses outside of yourself. OWN THEM!

We're all empowered to make our own decisions, and tuning into your internal world can make this truth real for you. Meditation can help you to gain a clearer perspective, and to call yourself out when you cast blame for your own self-sabotaging choices. If you're living on fast food because you swear you don't have time to prepare fresh, whole-food meals, you've validated your decision to remain unhealthy. Staying on this path reinforces the sense that health and fitness are not really your responsibility, and that you are powerless.

When you tell yourself these lies, the bottom line is that you are choosing a *why not* instead of a *why*. You're wasting your energy on the negative instead of the positive. And if you're not making choices that stem from your *why* in life, then ask yourself: Who are you making these choices for? Whose dreams are you supporting? What results are you working toward?

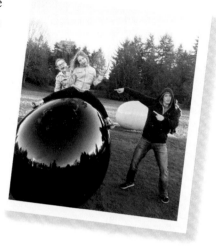

When life goes sideways and you physically can't make it to the gym, that doesn't mean you can't work out or move your body with purpose. Heck, no! You are your own best piece of gym equipment. Not only is your body free to use, but it's nearly always available to you. Even if you are dealing with an injury, you can modify your movements so you can still work out. As long as you have a body, and you have the ability to move, you can exercise. BAM*!*

Kids should be the motivation why we want to be fit and not the excuse why we can't.

THE *NO WILLPOWER* EXCUSE

I hear a lot of people complain that they have no willpower. They tell me, "I want to work out but I always give up because I'm just too weak (willed)." I counter this excuse by telling people to find something that they enjoy doing, and then really feed their connection to that activity. You have to start by identifying your desires. Not every exercise will be right for you, but keep trying different things to see what you like. Think of it this way: You never have to find the willpower to indulge in something that you love, such as getting a massage, or laughing with friends!

Of course, working out takes more effort than getting a massage, especially at the beginning when you haven't yet made it a habit. One way to help with motivation is to find someone to work out with, to be accountable to. Joining a fitness-based community is a great way to source allies who can support you. We motivate each other, and celebrate our personal victories together. The idea is to hold one another to a certain standard and ensure that you follow through to reach a goal.

What if every single person you know is overweight and complacent, and nobody wants to work out with you? No problem! Through social media, I can connect you with some fantastic online communities, where there are both private and public fitness groups. Not only can we see what the other members are doing, we can also encourage and support each other. Members post recipes, inspirational video and audio clips, share struggles, console and uplift one another, and act as sources of accountability, which we all need from time to time. It's all in the name of motivational

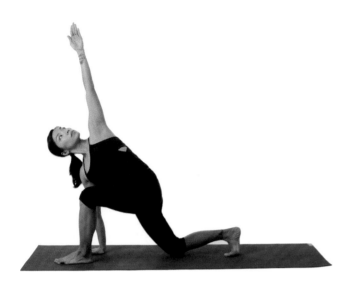

You can work out in a space as small as a yoga mat.

fun. There are also some engaging online tools, such as MyFitnessPal.com, and activity trackers, such as Fitbit, to help you gauge your progress against your health and fitness goals.

THE *NO SPACE* EXCUSE

I don't care how small your home is, it's big enough for you to work out in. All you really need is a space the size of, say, a bath towel, a yoga mat, or even a door-mat. You essentially want to create a little space for squats, push-ups, sit-ups, jogging on the spot and air skips. I'll describe these and other exercises in more detail in Chapter 7.

If you're a person who spends a lot of time on the road, I challenge you to never see this as a disruption to your fitness routine again. Most hotel rooms have a chair and a table, which you can use to create a mini-circuit for a 15-minute workout. You can even use the space between the wall and the bed. If you're a regular traveller, you probably know your itinerary in advance; that is, you don't likely just wake up in the morning and remember: *Oh, I have to head to San Francisco today.* So take a little time to plan for your health needs, and set yourself up to make good choices while you travel. This means carrying extra water (air travel can cause dehydration) and pack some healthy snacks, such as nuts and dried fruit. Remember that dehydration can be confused with hunger, so we often reach for the wrong foods when we're groggy after a flight. Above all, try to resist the lure of aimless channel surfing on the bed in your hotel room. Try to get out for a quick run in your host city instead. Fifteen minutes is all you need. You can do it!

THE *EVERYBODY ELSE COMES FIRST* EXCUSE

Too many of us simply don't prioritize our own health and fitness. When everybody around us seems to need something from us, putting our needs on the table can feel selfish—we may even feel guilty for doing something just for ourselves. Well, I'll be the first one to let you know that it's okay to look after *you*. In fact, you'll be better able to serve others by serving yourself first. When you understand and appreciate that, it puts your health into a different context. That is, neglecting your own health affects

BEWARE THE "SITTING DISEASE"!

Sitting is the new smoking! The more you sit, the more your health will suffer.

We love to sit—in our car, at the desk, on the couch, and at the game. New research shows that sitting and inactivity are linked to increased risks of heart disease, diabetes, cancer, and depression. Stated simply, our bodies are designed to move. A recent study showed that if we spent less than three hours a day sitting, our life expectancy would increase by two years. Furthermore, reducing TV time to less than two hours per day can increase your life expectancy by 1.4 years. That's a total of 3.4 years more of your life just by not sitting so much! Does that not make you want to stand up and read this book while pacing in your room? Do it now!

When I first started reading up on inactivity, and especially, the amount of time North Americans spend sitting, I immediately bought a standing desk. In fact, much of this book was written while I stood at my desk.

When you sit for long periods, your body adapts to the reduced physical demand by slowing down your metabolism. This means you burn fewer calories, and that extra energy is stored as fat.

Men who sit more than six hours a day have an 18 per cent increased risk of dying from heart disease and a 7.8 per cent increased chance of dying from diabetes, compared to someone who sits for three hours or less per day.

Today's North American 10-year-olds are the first generation expected to have a shorter life expectancy than their parents.

According to the American Medical Association, just 150 minutes of moderate exercise per week on-going is enough to drastically reduce the risk of sedentary lifestyle illnesses, such as obesity, diabetes, and heart disease.

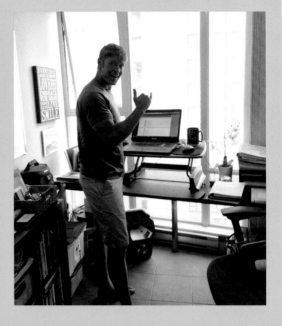

Globally, 20 per cent of early deaths are preventable with moderate exercise. And for the first time in history, inactivity-related illnesses killed 5.3 million people worldwide, more than smoking. Many health experts are thinking of inactivity as an illness, with some doctors in the U.S. pushing to make lack of exercise a medical diagnosis.

In the U.S., adults sit for an average of 8–10 hours each day. This makes the American lifestyle one of the most sedentary in the world. After long commutes and hours at our desks, we can hardly blame ourselves for taking a load off, but getting more exercise is a lot easier than most of us think.

everybody you care about, and not in a good way. You owe it to yourself to be healthy, but you also owe it to those who are closest to you, and they should understand that.

When we're not busy attending to our family's needs we're often at the beck and call of our employers. Perhaps you're a person who thinks, *I can't take time for myself because my career demands so much of me*. It's true that getting the right work/life balance can be tricky, but short-changing ourselves where our health is concerned never pays off. Poor health can take a terrible toll on your job performance and career.

The workforce has changed since the 1960s. Back then, nearly 50 per cent of private sector (non-government) jobs, such as construction, freight logistics and retail, required at least moderate-intensity physical activity. Currently, less than 20 per cent of jobs demand this level of activity. The average workweek is now longer, too. Full-time employees work an average of 47 hours per week, or 7 hours more per week than the standard 40-hour workweek. That translates to approximately 14 extra days of work per year, at jobs that are largely inactive!

> In this day and age, true role models are hard to find. Dai Manuel is a man who one can look up to and relate to. He wasn't born with a six-pack; he created it himself. He genuinely wants you to be the best version of yourself, in every aspect of your life. Dai and his wife are perfect examples of people living their lives to their potential and they inspire you to do the same. That's a role model."
>
> —BRITTANY

Additionally, employees now burn 100 fewer calories per workday than they did in the 1960s. A recent study, which compared workers from 1960 to 1962 with workers of 2003 to 2006, found that on average, employees are 17 pounds heavier than the average employee in the 1960s.

To add insult to injury, the past 50 years has seen the daily caloric intake increase by about 400 calories. This is a 20 per cent increase over the 1970 average, which hovered around 2,100 calories per day.

The bottom line is we're moving less and burning fewer calories, but we're eating more! And we wonder why we have an obesity epidemic on our hands?!

Surprisingly, the number one health issue in the workforce today isn't inactivity or obesity. It's stress. As you can imagine, inactivity and stress, coupled with longer working hours, has a massive impact on society. In fact, it's believed that lost productivity due to chronic pain amounts to $11.6 to $12.8 billion per year! And, hello, this one really gets to me, given my past: In the U.S., overweight or obese workers who have other chronic health problems miss about 450 million more days of work per year than healthy workers, costing more than $153 billion per year in lost productivity.

I can't emphasize this enough: Overwork and inactivity are disservices to your career *and* your employer. Is it any wonder that many corporations are investing millions of dollars into corporate wellness programs? They have learned that employee wellness affects the bottom line, both in hard costs and productivity. Good health means a happier, more satisfied workforce, which translates into increased productivity.

LETTING GO OF YOUR WHY NOTS

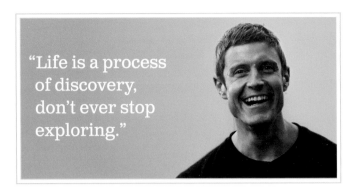

"Life is a process of discovery, don't ever stop exploring."

Years ago, I sustained an injury to my back during a competition. My L4-L5 vertebrae suffered a micro-tear, which caused a disc to protrude and pinch a nerve. It was one of the most excruciating injuries I've ever experienced. Up to that point I had only experienced mild pain from "throwing my back out" or overdoing it at the gym, but this injury gave me a whole new perspective on injuries involving nerves and other soft tissues. I wouldn't wish an experience like this on anyone.

I went through a period of self-doubt and formed a number of excuses about why I couldn't train anymore. "I'm hurt. I can't move right. I can't do what I was doing before, so why bother?" These were just a few of the mantras I repeated to myself during those first few weeks after getting hurt. I had a really hard time accepting that I would have to change the way I moved my body. I was quite rooted in how I trained, so the idea of modification didn't fit in my world.

This went on for nearly a month. I felt lethargic and heavy, and was putting myself down at every opportunity. I was drowning in my *poor me* monologue.

Thankfully, my wife Christie, being the feisty ginger that she is, called me out on my self-pity. She told me to get up and move, to stop feeling sorry for myself and to start adapting to my situation. (She's a wise one, isn't she?)

Adaptation is important, and accepting the need for adaptation is arguably even more important. It's challenging to overcome old habits that are entrenched. But I did exactly what Christie said, and started doing what I could. When I exercised, I focused on more isolated movements—nothing explosive or dynamic—and worked on re-stabilizing my core and the erector muscles that surround my spine. It was a slow process, but over time, I got stronger. I was training again and feeling great for it. This experience taught me a lot about myself, but even more about how to coach my clients.

When I begin working with new clients, I always ask them, "What do you need to release in order to do what you want to do?" This helps people to explore what's holding them back from becoming more fit. I meet most of the responses I get with a smirk,

GET A BIG HAIRY AUDACIOUS GOAL!

If you aren't ready to make this commitment to yourself, stop reading now; if you are, read on!

We all need goals.

I don't believe they define who we are, but they certainly say a lot about our character. Do you fumble through life and its challenges, or do you take control of your opportunities and set your sights on things outside of your grasp? I believe YOU to be the latter.

What's that one thing you've always wanted to do? You know, that one thing that you always tell yourself: One day I'm going to do that? And what's holding you back from going for it?

It's time to get going!

I urge my clients to Get a BHAG!, which stands for Big Hairy Audacious Goal. This is a term popularized by Jim Collins and Jerry I. Porras in their bestselling book Built to Last: Successful Habits of Visionary Companies. They describe a BHAG as a huge and powerful vision that an entire organization can rally around. I believe BHAGs aren't just for companies, but for individuals, too. That's why I urge my clients to set their sights on a huge challenge at least three to six months out. Committing yourself to this kind of goal can work as your why in the short-term.

Doing this is awesome for a number of reasons:

1. **Practicality.** It keeps you focused on the daily habits you need to adopt, and the steps you need to take, to make sure you arrive at your destination.
2. **Accountability.** Declaring your commitment is great for helping you stick to it.
3. **Discipline.** In challenging situations we have two choices: either give up or push through and conquer.

You like to win; I know you do. It's part of being human.

Over the years, I've used the following BHAGs to help my clients challenge themselves.

Every single person who finishes Tough Mudder feels an incredible sense of accomplishment. One of our I Want My Mudder teammates, Hersh, completed the course in just under seven hours. Did I mention that Hersh had a prosthetic leg? If Hersh could complete the course, I know that EVERYONE can do it.

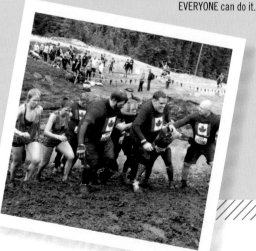

5 Big Hairy Audacious Goals You Want To Own

» **My First 5K:** I'm not a huge fan of running (heck, my nickname is Moose because I run like one), but I do get out for a few fun runs each year. Colour runs are a great place to start; why not check one out?

» **5K Mud Run:** Take the fun of a 5K to a team obstacle course in the mud. Mud runs have become wildly popular worldwide. A great example is the Spartan Race (see www.spartan.com). You might also want to check out my blog (www.daimanuel.com) for some cool videos and articles on mud runs, to see if this is something to put on your fitness goal list this year. Do it on your own, or better yet, recruit some friends and get after it.

» **A Mini-Triathlon:** Hey! I'm not saying you should register for an Ironman event. But I know if you were to commit to participating in a mini-tri six months out, you'd be ready by race day. It consists of a 750-metre (half-mile) swim, a 20-km (12-mile) bike ride, and a 5-km (3.1-mile) run. Don't be intimidated! It will be over before you know it, and six months is plenty of time to prep for this type of event, no matter your fitness level.

» **A Great Cause:** What better motivation than to commit to a fitness event for charity? I've been involved with the Grind for Kids charity for four years, which gets my team hiking the Grouse Grind, a 2.9-km trail straight up Grouse Mountain in my home city of Vancouver, all summer. The event raises money for the British Columbia Children's Hospital. Awesomeness! What local charities can you support by participating in a fitness event? Check one out, commit, and feel even more AWESOME for getting healthy and fit.

» **Tough Mudder:** This one is near and dear to my heart. Tough Mudder is a challenging 18- to 20-km (10- to 12-mile) outdoor obstacle course designed to test mental strength and physical grit. Having had the opportunity to lead a team (I Want My Mudder) over the last few years, I can honestly say that it's a life-changing event. No teammate is left behind!

So don't wait. What's your big hairy audacious fitness goal going to be?

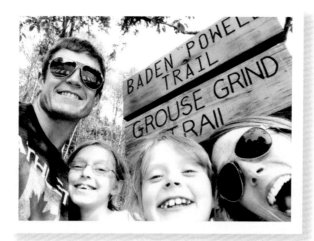

because many new clients say that they are prepared to cut back on TV, eat less garbage, and wake up 30 minutes earlier to get their Whole Life Fitness Power 30 done before work. This is commitment to a choice that must be put into action every single day. So of course I then ask, "Are you sure?" Because if there's any doubt, then the client may not have really identified the underlying *why* that will motivate them to fully commit to their decision to change.

Once you've completely realized your *why*—and owned it—it will be far easier to let go of your excuses because you simply can't kid yourself anymore. When you fully commit yourself to a goal—for example, wanting to be healthy enough to travel at 65—then it's easy to ditch any roadblocks that are standing in your way.

REALISTIC EXPECTATIONS, SUSTAINABLE RESULTS

I've seen too many people struggle to adopt a sustainable fitness plan because they have unreasonable expectations of what they think is required of them. They think they need to obsessively commit to fitness and hook up to highly ambitious programs.

> "If you really want to do something, you'll find a way. If you don't, you'll find an excuse."
>
> —JIM ROHN

Nothing could be further from the truth. The fact is we all have busy lives. Only professional athletes can work hours of cardio, strength training and conditioning into their everyday routine, because it's their job to do so. You do not have to reinvent your lifestyle in order to accommodate a new fitness regime, because that is simply not sustainable.

For example, I remember my good friend Jon, who was excited about his newly purchased DVD fitness program. He was committed to making it work for him and was sure he could adopt it into his everyday routine. Jon is married, works 50 hours a week and has children, along with coaching commitments. Jon was struggling to maintain his relationship with his wife, as the only time they saw each other was on weekends and evenings after the kids went to bed. But he was sure that he could fit in an extra six to eight hours a week to work the fitness program. And you know what happened? The DVDs were shelved after day four, and haven't seen the light of day since.

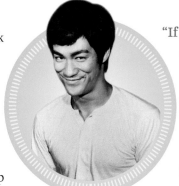

"If you always put limits on everything you do, physical or [otherwise], it will spread into your work and [other areas of] your life. There are no limits. There are only plateaus, and you must not stay there; you must go beyond them." —BRUCE LEE

It would be far better for someone like Jon to take a step back and look at their actual lifestyle as it stands, and evaluate where there's time to work in some more health and fitness. In other words, it is much easier and makes more sense to find a fitness program that fits our lifestyle, than to overhaul our lifestyle to fit a fitness program. If you want to be diligent and follow through on your fitness goals, it's crucial to start off with a sustainable plan.

Personally, early morning workouts are what work best for me. Five-thirty a.m. is *my* time. I developed the habit of getting going early back when I was teaching classes and personal training sessions; now, I try to stick with that routine as often as possible. But I understand that 5:30 a.m. is not a fit for everybody. Throughout the day, we all have our peaks and valleys, from an energy standpoint, so you'll need to figure out what makes sense for you.

Find something that can fit into your routine. Walk to the park, either by yourself or with your family or a friend. Walk your kids to school, or pick them up. Just start making little decisions to get moving. Remember that you will not suddenly have more hours in the day. Your life will have exactly the same amount of time as before, but now your health has become a priority and you're doing what you need to do to improve it. Everybody can do that.

Essentially, giving the boot to your *why nots* means showing up in your life to a new degree. The simple act of removing your obstacles in support of your health works a mental muscle that gets stronger the more you use it. You'll find that eventually, it will become second nature to you to remove obstacles and excuses in other areas of your life, too.

While the excuses in this chapter are the most common ones I have come across in my career, there are an infinite number of others. We all have challenges and mental crutches, but with courage and dedication, you can move through them.

So, are you with me?

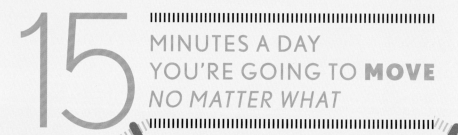

15 MINUTES A DAY
YOU'RE GOING TO **MOVE**
NO MATTER WHAT

This is a **FOREVER** piece

this is a *lifestyle*

It will have a **CASCADING** effect

Own your **CHOICES**

It's **TIME** to be the **CHANGE AGENTS** in our lives

You can accomplish **A LOT** by doing **A LITTLE** training **EVERY DAY**

31

EVERY **LITTLE ACTION** BUILDS INTO A **BIGGER RESULT**

IT'S ABOUT TIME

WHAT WOULD YOU SAY IS the one biggest hurdle that prevents you from leading a more consistently active life? Is it that you're travelling, raising a family, perhaps working at a busy job?

I've got news for you. All of these seemingly different excuses are just versions of one thing: a big old time crunch. We're all strapped for time, for a million different reasons. In our whiplash-paced society, it's little wonder that there's one heck of a widespread perception that we don't have time to work out.

Our days are limited to 24 hours, of which one third is spent sleeping (if you're lucky) and, for many of us, at least another third is spent doing a job that is often stressful and largely sedentary.

To make your head spin, here are some statistics about time:

1. The *American Journal of Epidemiology* estimates that the average American spends 55 per cent of waking time (7.7 hours per day) in sedentary behaviours such as sitting.

2. A 13-year-long study published in 2010 by the American Cancer Society found that women who sat for more than six hours per day were 37 per cent more likely to die during the time period studied than those who sat for fewer than six hours per day. The study also showed that men who sat for over six hours a day were 18 per cent more likely to die during the study period.

   Those who were long-time sitters and also generally inactive in their day to day lives had even higher mortality rates during the study period: 94 and 48 per cent for women and men, respectively.

3. According to The Nielsen Corporation, the average American watches more than four hours of TV each

> "Dai has taught me that although life is busy there is always enough time in a day to dedicate to ME! I deserve it! On the other hand, he has also taught me not to beat myself up if there is a day here and there that I cannot do that. That's life! I can honestly say I love the person I am becoming more and more every day, thanks to Dai and Christie!"
> —CARMEN

day (or 28 hours/week, or two months of nonstop TV-watching per year). In a 65-year life, that person will have spent nine years glued to the tube. Canadians are similar, clocking in a whopping average of 30 hours of TV viewing a week. (Compare that to the following mind-blowing stat: The average time that Canadian parents spend engaged in meaningful conversation with their child is only 3.5 minutes per week!)

4. The World Health Organization published the following statistics about physical activity (stand up to read this one):

   a. Insufficient physical activity is one of the ten leading risk factors for death worldwide. People who are insufficiently active have a 20 to 30 per cent increased risk of death compared to people who are sufficiently active.

   b. Insufficient physical activity is a key risk factor for non-communicable diseases (NCDS) such as cardiovascular diseases, cancer and diabetes.

   c. Physical activity has significant health benefits and contributes toward preventing NCDS.

   d. Globally, one in four adults are not getting the recommended minimum of 150 minutes of moderate-intensity or 75 minutes of vigorous-intensity physical activity per week.

   e. More than 80 per cent of the world's adolescent population is insufficiently physically active.

> " **Those who think they have no time for healthy eating will sooner or later have to find time for illness** "
>
> —EDWARD STANLEY

As a society, we are moving less and eating more. We live in a culture of instant gratification. We consume calories on autopilot, and get into our cars to travel two blocks. Collectively, we are getting more and more out of shape. Today, a state of poor health (or as I like to say, "*un*-health") feels more "normal" to many of us than being healthy does. The biggest problem is that when you don't even know what you're missing, it's pretty hard to imagine a better way.

The hard truth is that when we don't make time for health, we will ultimately have to make time for disease and illness.

Reminders that time is fleeting surround us. The late Apple founder Steve Jobs stated during his famous address to the 2005 graduating class of Stanford University, "Remembering that I'll be dead soon is the most important tool I've ever encountered to help me make the big choices in life." Essentially, Jobs was saying that accepting the fact that you're eventually going to die allows you the mental freedom to design a life that is awesome.

We can all be the change agents in our own lives. Right now, in this moment, you can choose to stop using lack of time as an excuse for inaction. Instead of saying, "Time owns me; I'm powerless over my own schedule," try saying, "Hello, Time, old friend. I've decided to get healthy." Try to see time as a positive force in your whole-life fitness, not a barrier to it.

BLOCK YOUR TIME

Sadly, we can't just buy time like a commodity. We can only work with what we've got, and that's not always easy. I get it. I've been there myself!

I came to a major turning point in my life when I realized that, although I might not be able to manage my time minute by minute, I can manage my commitments by blocking off chunks of time for the things that matter to me. If it's not blocked out on my calendar, the likelihood of it happening decreases. Of course, everyone uses a calendar to keep track of appointments, but I'm talking about scheduling those regular, recurring commitments that fill our days, such as working, running errands and spending quality time with family. By visualizing my commitments as blocks of time and mapping them out across a weekly agenda, I can turn time into a tangible thing that I can see and have greater control over. To work fitness into your life on a regular basis, schedule it—and stick to it.

I encourage my clients to print out an agenda every week, and block out all the activities they know they have to commit to doing, from bringing children home from school, to attending a night-school class or volunteer sessions. Be realistic about how long these activities or commitments take (and don't forget to include the journey there and back). Add your work commitments—again, including your commute, if you have one.

Once you've blocked out your commitments, really look at the shape of your days and week, and ask yourself: *Where can I fit in my daily commitment to myself?* And yes, it has to be daily, or close to it. As you know by now, I'm a big believer in trying to move your body every day, because a body at rest likes to stay at rest. If you let your body do nothing, it's going to be more than happy to continue to do nothing.

Block out time for your health and stick to it.

WHEN WILL YOU FIT ACTIVITY INTO YOUR DAY?	MORNING	AFTERNOON	EVENING
Monday			
Tuesday			
Wednesday			
Thursday			
Friday			
Saturday			
Sunday			

But let's get one thing straight: that daily time commitment doesn't have to be huge. Many people overestimate what's required, especially when it comes to making New Year's resolutions. Starting January 1, you see the "resolutionists" committing to grueling 90-minute workouts at the gym four times a week, and swearing that this is the year they're going to do it.

But the truth is, this is probably too much for most people to sustain, and the trouble may be twofold. First, it's a shock to the system. Strength and endurance need to be built gradually, so propelling yourself from the couch to extreme workout programs isn't good for you. Second, it's hard on your motivation. What's more defeating than falling at the first hurdle, failing to keep your date with the gym come February?

The problem comes from the mistaken belief that you need to reinvent your lifestyle to fit in these extra hours at the gym. Resolutionists who try to do this often don't think about the extra steps that have to be factored in to make their promise a reality. Spending four evenings a week at the gym likely means they have to let something else go in order to fit that into their schedule. There's a reason why it didn't work before, right? To think that they're miraculously going to cram it all in without compromising other commitments is unrealistic, and it can be very discouraging, too.

> "The Whole Life Fitness Power 30 helped me get motivated and stay true to my training and self-development. I felt energized and confident during the program and can't wait to use the tools Dai and Christie have given me to keep bettering myself. Thirty minutes a day for yourself—everyone can do it!" —CAITLIN

THE CROSSFIT CROSSOVER

Like every parent, my world changed when I became a father. Suddenly, my time was not mine alone, but also my daughters'. I wanted to spend every moment with them. What's not to love about watching a child's miraculous development? I wanted to be with them for every great milestone—their first smiles, their first chuckles, their first words.

However, I knew I had to balance this love-fest with my fitness, and at first, I didn't handle it well at all. I was in the midst of building my fitness retail business, logging 50 to 60 hours per week, trying to maintain a baseline level of health and fitness, and on top of that, trying to be a great father and husband. Knowing that my health and fitness was still a priority to me, I would spend an hour or so at the gym after work, which was actually a two-hour time commitment (or more) after factoring in the commute and shower time (and of course conversations around the water fountain). This wasn't sustainable because I felt guilty for not being home with my family, and I was missing out on important moments with them. Having spoken about this with my coaching clients, I know that this is common for many people.

My life was revolutionized at the age of 30 when I was introduced to a then-new exercise concept called CrossFit, which showed me how to achieve and maintain a high level of fitness in very little time.

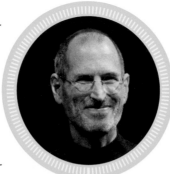

"Remembering that I'll be dead soon is the most important tool I've ever encountered to help me make the big choices in life."—STEVE JOBS

Typical gym workouts include long sessions consisting mostly of weight training with a little cardio. My typical split during the week would see me spend an hour on my back and chest one day, triceps and biceps the next, followed by legs, with an abs day thrown in here and there. I'd also have days dedicated to cardio and core, spending 45 to 50 minutes focusing on burning calories and getting my heart rate elevated for a sustained period of time. All in all, my gym routine usually took from seven to 10 hours per week.

There are many things to consider when it comes to exercising, or "moving with purpose," as I like to call it. I will always recommend incorporating full-body workouts, focusing on aspects such as balance, agility, coordination and other skills that round out your fitness. But trying to work all of these aspects into your routine requires a lot of planning and knowledge, which often leads to routines that are so complicated that you spend more time trying to understand the exercises than actually doing them.

CrossFit is different. It incorporates the principle of efficient movement, mindfully done. That is, instead of lengthy weight and cardio training circuits, CrossFit workouts introduced me to a training method known as an AMRAP, which stands for *as many reps as possible*, or, *as many rounds as possible*. It means working out at a sustained level of intensity for a set period of time without stopping. In any given workout, you might do only a few movements, but you're constantly in motion until your time is up. As you become healthier and fitter, you can increase your time limit or keep it the same, but the workload and intensity will gradually change. Your capacity will increase and you'll find that you're doing more reps or more rounds in that same block of time.

I found that this new way of working out—doing a short and intense workout every day—made great sense for my body. It also made sense for my life, which suffers the same time crunch that others face. The principles of CrossFit allow me to take care

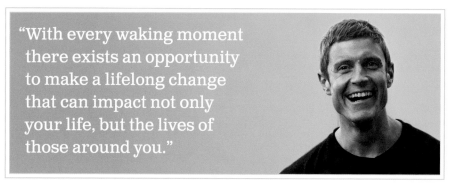

of my fitness needs quickly, so I can devote adequate time to my other Fs: Family, Finances, Faith and Fun.

In other words, you can accomplish a *lot* by doing a *little* training every day. You just need to make sure that the "little" is well designed, attuned to your goals, and power-packed.

I base all of my programs on these principles, which is why Whole Life Fitness Power 30 workouts can be completed in just 15 minutes. It might be hard to believe that's all it takes to get fit, but I find that it is ideal, not only because it's effective but also because it is sustainable. Everybody has 15 minutes! I don't care who you are, what you do, or what kind of life you live; I can find 15 minutes in your day for a quick workout.

Once you get going, you'll see how making your workout commitment manageable will help you to seamlessly integrate fitness into your life. For 15 minutes a day, you're going to move, no matter what. This works out to almost one per cent of a 24-hour day. Isn't that a worthwhile way to spend *one per cent* of your time? If you really want to go for the gold in your own life, you might choose to follow your daily workout with 15 minutes of meditation and personal development. And why not? That would still amount to only two per cent of your 24-hour day.

Of course, there's always an opportunity to do more. I encourage my clients to be active throughout the day, for example, by parking as far from the store as possible in the grocery store parking lot, by taking the stairs instead of the elevator, by doing some extra movements in the park while your kids are playing, by clenching your glutes while you're sitting at your desk, or by going for an energetic walk during your lunch break rather than shooting the breeze by the water cooler. It all adds up!

This is not a fad; it's a lifestyle. It's a forever habit. Making this kind of sustained commitment to your own health and well-being will have a massive effect on your entire life that will play out in everything you do.

MOVE OVER, TIME VAMPIRES

Once you start examining how and where you spend your time, you'll soon notice a whole range of "time vampires" that rise up to suck the time right out of your day. Very often, you don't even feel them doing it!

Maybe watching television is a big time vampire for you, or catching up on social media, or playing video games. If screens demand a lot of your attention, you're not alone: Americans spend more than nine times as many minutes watching television or movies as they do on sports and exercise, according to research conducted by the University of California. The Bureau of Broadcast Measurement Canada reports that the average Canadian adult watches 30 hours of TV every week. Other time vampires that might be sinking their teeth into your schedule include drinking, gossiping or simply putzing around aimlessly, whiling away time without any purpose. We've all got our weaknesses when it comes to wasting time, and they show up in many different ways.

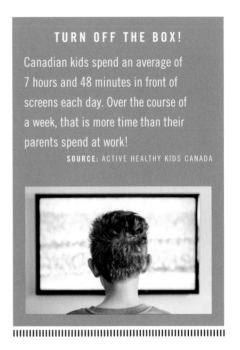

TURN OFF THE BOX!

Canadian kids spend an average of 7 hours and 48 minutes in front of screens each day. Over the course of a week, that is more time than their parents spend at work!

SOURCE: ACTIVE HEALTHY KIDS CANADA

The question is, just how can you steal your time back from those vampires? It starts with prioritizing your health and long-term happiness.

Whether your ideal window is in the morning, afternoon or evening, the main thing is just to find those 15 minutes for physical activity and 15 minutes for personal development. You don't have to take it from your kids. You don't have to take it from your job. You don't have to take it from your parents. But maybe you can take it from TV, Facebook, or any other activity that drains hours from your life without paying you back with lasting well-being.

If you're a hockey, football, or *MasterChef* fan, I'm not going to tell you that you shouldn't indulge in your passion. But maybe you can find creative ways to allow your pastimes to support your health rather than undermine it. There are always breaks in gameplay, not to mention commercial breaks during TV shows. Those can add up to a decent chunk of time over the course of a game or program. I challenge you to use those minutes to do something physical in front of the TV. By dovetailing your fitness into another activity that you already love to do, you set off a positive cascading effect in which one thing reinforces the other.

FIVE POSITIVE WAYS TO MANAGE YOUR STRESS

Many people revert to unhealthy methods of stress busting, which may offer temporary relief but do very little to reduce stress in the long term. Some can even be harmful. I'm talking about substance abuse, smoking, venting to others, playing video games, or zoning out in front of the TV.

The good news is that there are many simple but healthy, effective ways of dealing with stress, but they may require you to change the way you think and behave. While some stressors are unavoidable, you can limit their ability to affect you negatively.

1. **STOP OVERCOMMITTING**
   Accept that you are not a superhuman. You can't do everything, and you can't always be perfect—what you might find surprising is that most people won't expect you to be. Try to be more assertive, and learn to say no!

2. **CONTROL YOUR ENVIRONMENT**
   The people we spend time with influence our thoughts and feelings. If you are finding that you are surrounded by naysayers, or people who are quick to find fault in everything you are doing or trying to change, it's time to re-evaluate your support network. You need an environment that is positive and encouraging. You need a tribe of people that say, "You can do it!" Stay away from negative people, especially if they drive you crazy!

3. **THINK POSITIVELY**
   Thinking positively is particularly difficult if you have a habit of being tough on yourself, or if you've fallen into the habit of being pessimistic. The key is to look for the good in everything that happens, rather than feeling as though the universe is conspiring against you at every turn. This takes effort, but like anything, the more you practise, the more familiar and easier it becomes. If you find that old, unresolved issues are bubbling to the surface, it will undoubtedly help to talk them out, so confide in a trusted loved one, or seek the help of a professional therapist.

4. **DO WHAT MAKES YOU HAPPY**
   One of the best ways to bust stress is to live in the moment, and to do the things you enjoy most. Play with your kids, go for a long walk, read a book, or listen to uplifting music. By making these life-enhancing activities a priority, you are telling yourself that your feelings matter! It's kind of like giving yourself a big hug.

5. **ADOPT A HEALTHY LIFESTYLE**
   Unhealthy lifestyles are hard on the body and the mind, and will inevitably exacerbate your stress levels. Strive instead to maximize your energy levels in every way. Ditch the junk food, caffeine, and sugar and go for fresh, home cooked meals and snacks. Avoid alcohol and drugs, which can numb you and drain your energy, even in low doses. Finally, be sure to get plenty of sleep. Tiredness makes us less resilient and more susceptible to feeling overwhelmed by negative emotions.

You might have heard of "gateway drugs," which can trigger the abuse of harder, even more addictive substances. Let's put a positive spin on that concept. Think about the Whole Life Fitness Power 30 as your "gateway fitness plan." Once you try it, hot damn, you'll be hooked! It will lead to more movement, extra workouts and more active participation in the world around you, perhaps through team sports or community events.

If you're like many of my clients, you will start to see your workout as a daily "reset." This is one of the biggest reasons why I love my 15-minute hit. Even on days when I can't get to the gym or find time for a long walk, my quick daily workout is always there for me and acts as a mental reset button. I always know that whatever else is going on in my day, I'll have a chance to burn off some steam and excess energy, and get focused. I inevitably feel better afterward. Who wouldn't look forward to that and want it in their life every day?

The second half of my Whole Life Fitness Power 30 routine, involving five minutes of mindfulness and 10 minutes of personal development, is when I fill my mind with a little positive juice. After a brief five-minute meditation, sometimes I'll read from an inspiring book. Other times I'll spend those minutes journaling. Documenting your thoughts like this is a great way to connect with yourself and anchor your goals. Spend some time reflecting on your thoughts, and write down what you discover. What are you doing in your daily life that makes you feel good? What would you like to do more of, and what would you like to move away from? Have you come across any positive messages in personal development books that resonate with you? Over time, you'll start to see how the ideas of the great thinkers in the world can be reflected on your own mental canvas and applied to your life.

Ten minutes of personal development per day effortlessly turns into 70 minutes a week, and 300 minutes (or five hours) a month. And then, BAM! After a year, you will have clocked two and a half days of personal development. Books will be read; journals will be filled. You'll have a whole pile of expressed words, thoughts better understood, and real insights gained for your precious time investment. Can I get a high-five on how awesome that is?

> "The daily 10 minutes of personal development has helped me rediscover a creative outlet that I enjoy. In sharing my thoughts and ideas with Dai and Christie through the Whole Life Fitness Power 30, I received heartwarming support. It has really gotten me out of my own way and to be open to more possibilities for myself than I ever imagined 30 days ago." —JANE

SHARE THE PASSION FOR **HEALTH**, **FITNESS**, **WELLNESS** AND **ACTIVE LIVING**, WELCOMING ALL LIKE-MINDED PEOPLE INTO **OUR TRIBE**.

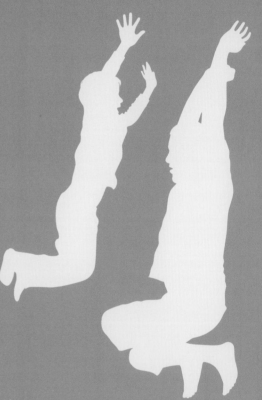

Because the Whole Life Fitness Power 30 is based on very compact chunks of time, it's always accessible to you, no matter what. You'll learn to never again use time as an excuse. You might not always choose to follow through with your plan. I get it; life happens. But that's really what I want to hammer home: You make the choice. It's up to you to own your situation. Own your choices. You can't blame time for your decisions, once you accept that you're the one who chooses what to do with it.

The result of committing 30 minutes each day to my own well-being is that I always feel like I've accomplished something. That time is my "win" of my day—and I'd love it to be yours, too. Life can be a journey of constant growth and self-improvement, and this routine is a rock solid tool that you can use to really make that happen—physically, emotionally and psychologically. Moment by moment, you will find that you feel just a little bit better than you did the day before, much better than you did a month ago, and a whole heck of a lot better than you did the year before.

Gradually, the Whole Life Fitness Power 30 will become a daily ritual that keeps you on track in every aspect of your life, a daily ritual you don't even think twice about. And it will have you laughing in the face of the words: *I don't have time.*

"Dai's influence was formidable. He was a prime motivator for me to quit smoking and evolve into a healthier lifestyle, become more productive as a CEO, and grow as an individual." —JEFF

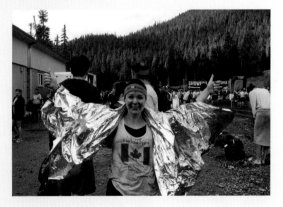

"The Whole Life Fitness program has been a process that has not only allowed me to get in the best shape of my life, it also has given me a focus that I've never had before. It encompasses not only physical fitness and health but also facing personal struggles and fears.

I started with Whole Life Fitness after struggling to get back into shape after having a baby. Dai challenged me to do Tough Mudder. The idea sounded insane to me! But not only was I ready for Tough Mudder, I loved it!

I'm a better person for being a part of this group and plan to continue with the patterns I have established through it." —BECKY

MINDFULNESS
is just like a muscle –
BUILD IT UP!

Take a **deep** breath

BROADEN YOUR **HORIZON**

Go with the *flow*

BE **KIND** TO YOURSELF

BE *in the* MOMENT

Quiet the voice inside you

YOU DESERVE **ALL THE HAPPINESS** IN THE WORLD

Tone your **mind**

STAY POSITIVE

MENTAL FITNESS

WHAT'S THE FIRST THING THAT comes to your mind when you think of meditation: Buddhist monks in saffron robes, cross-legged yogis, or modern spiritual seekers? No doubt there's some truth in all of these clichés, but these days it's not only monks and religious devotees who are enthusiastic meditators.

My first introduction to mindful action was Mr. Miyagi's mesmerizing voice saying to Daniel-san, "Wax on, wax off…" Joking aside, I was transfixed by *The Karate Kid* as a child. Here was a young teen wanting nothing more than to learn to fight to defend himself. But with the guidance of his sensei Mr. Miyagi, he not only learned to defend himself, but also to quiet his mind and focus on a single action, through the practise of karate.

Now, with the incredible growth in the popularity of yoga and other mindful practices, meditation has gone mainstream. People from all walks of life are discovering the benefits of going within as part of a healthy lifestyle. No more are my trademark "BAM!" and "HOORAH!" enough. I think I need to start introducing new mantras like "OM." And I love it!

Paradoxically, stillness is one of the most important aspects of the Whole Life Fitness Power 30. After regular exercise, a healthy diet and good sleep habits, calming the mind is one of the best possible ways to support the body. (And honestly, it is one of the things I struggle with most.)

Daily meditation practice tunes up your brain, enhancing mental and physical well-being and reducing chronic pain and stress. Clinical trials have shown that mindfulness can conveniently and effectively replace painkillers. In a randomized controlled clinical trial, researchers studied 109 patients with varying levels of chronic pain. Some were placed in

> " Normally at the end of the night I liked to watch TV, which was accompanied by junk food. Since I started doing the 10 minutes of self-development, instead I find myself watching tons of TED Talks, watching tutorials on how to further my business, and finding out what's going on in other parts of the world. The '10 minutes' turned into an hour or more. Now I have more to talk about with people other than what happened on *The Bachelorette* last night. Strangely, this particular personal development has me holding my head higher than ever."
> —MARIA

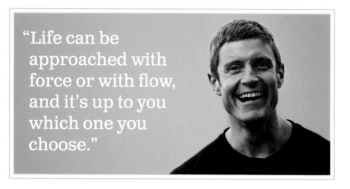

"Life can be approached with force or with flow, and it's up to you which one you choose."

mindfulness-based stress reduction programs, and the remainder were placed in a control group. The results were amazing! The group utilizing meditation as a form of pain management experienced a reduction in general anxiety and depression, an improved sense of mental well-being, and reported feeling more in control of their pain, along with having higher pain acceptance. Sure beats popping a pill, doesn't it? Studies have also found that daily meditation can reduce the risk of developing cardiovascular disease. And lastly, mind-body medicine through meditative practice has been shown to boost the more conventional treatments of cancer, high blood pressure, asthma, obesity, pain and nausea, insomnia, diabetes, mental health issues and fibromyalgia. Although meditation alone can't guarantee specific medical results, I can tell you from my own experience and through working with clients that reducing your stress (and stress hormones) will have a positive effect on many aspects of your life.

It's not always easy to find a moment of calm, especially for those of us living in busy cities, where we're under constant pressure. But just like a pressure cooker, we need to find a way to let off some steam. Like many others, I used to look to food and drink as a way to deal with stress. Eating sweets releases feel-good endorphins to surge through your body, but the effect is short-lived. Alcohol may seem to bring short-term relief from stress, but is actually a depressant that slows down reaction time, impairs vision and makes it harder to think clearly. Over time, alcohol abuse can have a negative impact on the liver and kidneys, and put you in a higher risk category for heart attack, stroke and various forms of cancer. In other words, these seemingly easy ways to deal with stress come at a cost.

As an overweight teen, I dealt with stress by absorbing myself in TV, video games and movies and by eating sweets and fatty foods. By focusing my attention on things outside of myself, I was able to pretend that all was okay for a brief moment. Whenever the stark reality of my situation hit me, I'd go back to grasping for the temporary high I got from the spike in my blood sugar.

At the time, I interpreted that feeling as happiness, but now that I have a better understanding of the connection between certain foods and depression, it's no wonder I felt as low as I did when I was in that state of self-prescribed numbness. The foods I ate were actually making me more depressed the more I ate them.

Have you ever noticed how you feel when eating a highly processed fast-food meal or baked treat that's loaded with refined sugar? I bet you felt pretty awesome while you were eating it—taste buds exploding, aromas triggering an uncontrollable salivary response, and to top it off, a pleasing texture hitting your tongue. In the words of Homer H. Simpson, it feels like: *Arghhhhhhhhh!* But as good as eating these treats might feel at the time, a 2012 study found that junk food consumption may increase a person's risk of developing depression. Luckily, there is a healthier route to relief from the stress of modern life, and it's available to all of us, all of the time.

GOING WITH THE FLOW

Life can be approached with force or with flow. Force is simple—it's what many of us do day-to-day without even realizing we're doing it. We jam our days full of activity and obligations, often over-committing ourselves, and then we spend the day stressing out about how we're going to make it work. When it gets to be too much to bear, we swear we won't do it again, but sure enough, we do it anyway. We force our schedules, we force our lifestyles, and we force ourselves to do things we don't want to do because we feel we ought to do them.

Any of this sound familiar? It's okay, we're friends; we can be candid and open with one another. As I have admitted, I lived the better part of my life this way, until I made some big changes a few years ago.

Flow, as it's known among psychology experts, is another state of being. Flow describes a mental state of complete focus and concentration; it happens when a person is fully immersed in the activity in which they're engaged. When we are in a state of flow, we are completely and utterly absorbed in what we are doing. Sounds pretty awesome, doesn't it?

According to positive psychologist Dr. Mihaly Csikszent-mihalyi, there are 10 factors that play into the experience of "flow". They are:

1. Clear goals, while challenging, are still attainable.
2. Strong concentration and focused attention.
3. The activity is intrinsically rewarding.
4. Feelings of serenity; a loss of feelings of self-consciousness.

> "If somebody had told me that 30 minutes a day would change my life I would have said they were ridiculous but the Whole Life Fitness Power 30 has changed my relationship with my body, my husband, my daughter, my work, my friends and family. It's just been amazing and I will never go back to how I was before. You are game changers." —JENN

5. Timelessness; a distorted sense of time; feeling so focused on the present that you lose track of time passing.
6. Immediate feedback.
7. Knowing that the task is doable; a balance between skill level and the challenge presented.
8. Feelings of personal control over the situation and the outcome.
9. Lack of awareness of physical needs.
10. Complete focus on the activity itself.

So I ask you, which approach would you ideally like to take in your life? I'm all about flow with intent. Being passionately aware of my life, relationships, my surroundings, and using all of my senses to fully experience my environment...now that's LIVING to the max.

Being in a state of forced living leaves you little time to "smell the roses," as they say. You're caught up in the hustle and bustle of life, being pulled in a hundred different directions. You feel the pressure of the high expectations you have set for yourself. Goals feel out of reach, and your life plan seems vague or, worse, unattainable.

But when you let yourself enter a state of *flow*, you'll soon find that your circumstances and surroundings seem to move into alignment with your intentions. Life simply starts falling into place.

Sounds surreal, doesn't it? I was definitely a naysayer at first, rejecting the very idea of mindfulness and meditation. But that changed when I decided to let go and give my life my full attention. Ask yourself one question: What's the worst thing that could happen if you gave yourself over to a daily habit involving mindfulness or meditation? I think you already know the answer. There's no downside to trying it, and so much to potentially gain.

We all know the perils of poor stress management, and how it feels when we are either obsessing about a past mistake, or worrying about the future. It can feel like a never-ending itch, and we just keep scratching it mentally. Scientist and author Kathryn Tristan exposes this kind of stress in her book, *Why Worry? Stop Coping and Start Living.* "Learning to live and appreciate the present moment is an antidote to stress," she writes, "But it also requires living mindfully and changing unproductive habits."

Jon Kabat-Zinn is the founder of the Stress Reduction Clinic and the Center for Mindfulness in Medicine, Health Care, and Society at the University of Massachusetts Medical School. In his book, *Full Catastrophe Living: Using the Wisdom of Your Body and Mind to Face Stress, Pain, and Illness*, he defines mindfulness as, "paying attention in a particular way. On purpose, in the moment, and non-judgmentally." He actively encourages his readers to build the habit of mindfulness into their daily routines to achieve bliss.

By paying attention to our lives non-judgmentally, mindfulness allows us to look at the bigger picture and stop torturing ourselves with a perceived sense of lack. Look, life's not perfect. We will never be happy if we keep focusing on what we are missing. But we can be content NOW with what we have. It helps to remember that satisfaction can't be measured in terms of material things. It needs to be felt from within—and that is always within our control.

Who hasn't experienced moments of heart-racing worry? That's unavoidable in our fast-paced world. The trouble comes when we get stuck overthinking a problem that doesn't have a productive outcome, or when we stress out about something that might never happen. This is a huge drain on your emotions, your energy and your ability to function productively.

The negative voice inside your head might be repetitive, loud, habitual and involuntary, but that doesn't mean you have to take it too seriously! The simple fact is, you will ultimately end up being ruled by your thoughts if you cannot take control of them. We *can't* control everything that happens to us, so it's okay to stop trying! You won't be comfortable all of the time in your life, but that's okay, too. Learning to live with a certain amount of discomfort, uncertainty, or even disappointment is key to finding peace of mind.

> "Your mind is at work all day, every day. Every decision you make, every challenge that you face, every moment you go through in life, your mind is your constant companion... and it can be your best friend or your worst enemy."
> —CHRISTOPHER LLOYD CLARKE, MUSICIAN

Be kind to yourself, because you deserve the love and kindness you give to others. In fact, you are worthy of all the happiness in the world! Try to remember that you are enough. Negative thoughts, self-pitying, and even doom and gloom will inevitably enter your mind from time to time, but you can learn to redirect your energy in a more positive direction.

MINDFULNESS IS MEDITATION

Mindfulness, in essence, is a very simple form of meditation. One of the most common ways to practise this is to concentrate on your breathing and focus your attention on the moment at hand. It's all about connecting to your inner self without judgment or criticism. Some people find it helpful to continuously repeat a specific phrase (or mantra) or closely focus on the sensation of your breath flowing in and out of your body, while allowing the free flow of thoughts to enter and leave your mind, without getting caught up in them.

Each of us has an endless parade of thoughts moving through our awareness. When we try to concern ourselves with each and every one, they can start to pile up like items on a factory line conveyor belt, just like in that famous chocolate-wrapping scene in *I Love Lucy*. When the conveyor belt becomes overburdened, it can lead to anxiety and even depression, getting in the way of our ability to pursue our goals productively. Just like Lucy, we get overwhelmed. We rush. We overcompensate. We panic. We cry.

So here's the thing: Thoughts and feelings change with each passing moment. It's within your power to decide which ones to pay attention to and which ones to

Life doesn't have to feel like a conveyor belt. You can learn to let those unhealthy thoughts go!

act upon. Without good mental self-management, we are at the mercy of whatever shows up in our awareness. But with mindful self-awareness, we can consciously choose how to respond to each thought; that is, whether to give it deeper consideration, to act on it, or, if it's an unhelpful or unhealthy thought, to simply let it go. Meditation allows you to practise letting go and letting your thoughts and feelings flow. As you calm your fight-or-flight response, you'll soon reduce your tendency to react to each and every thought. Thoughts will still enter your mind as they did before, but you'll learn to let them burst like soap bubbles when they aren't the thoughts that you want to have.

LET'S GET STARTED

Maybe you have experienced moments of soul searching, in which you connected with your inner self and reflected on your life. If so, you've already taken a step toward basic meditation principles. There is more than one way to practise mindfulness, but the goal is ultimately to achieve a state of mind that is relaxed and focused at the same time. As author and mindfulness expert Ed Halliwell says, "It's only when we meditate for its own sake—rather than trying to get something from it—that we find the results we're after."

> "Do not dwell in the past, do not dream of the future, concentrate the mind on the present moment."—BUDDHA

Here are some techniques to try.

- **Basic mindfulness meditation:** Sit quietly and focus on your natural breath, or on a word or mantra that you repeat silently. Allow thoughts to come and go without judgment, gently returning your focus to your breath or mantra.
- **Body sensations:** Notice subtle body sensations, such as an itch or tingling, without judgment and let them pass (well, if you really *have* to scratch that itch, just do so, then get back to meditating). Do a mental scan of your body, from head to toe, taking note of the sensations throughout your body.
- **Sensory:** Notice what you see, hear, smell, taste and touch. Whether you are active in a seated, walking or eating meditation, silently name them "sight," "sound," "smell," "taste," or "touch" and then let them go.
- **Emotions:** Allow emotions to be present without judgment. Practise a steady and relaxed naming of emotions: "joy," "anger," "frustration." Accept the presence of your emotions without judgment and let them go.
- **Urge surfing:** Cope with cravings (for addictive substances or behaviours) and allow them to pass. Notice how your body feels as the craving enters. Replace the craving with the knowledge that it will eventually subside.

When you meditate, the important thing is in trying to allow your mind to roam freely, thoughts floating to the surface of your awareness without judgment. In this state, you are free from the tensions, worries and priorities of life, and you can truly live in the moment. You might experiment with reflecting on your personality, your

> "I looked at my pictures pre- and post-Whole Life Fitness Power 30 and was struck not only by my loss of weight but how my posture had changed. It is not just because of the physical aspect of committing to a daily workout, but to the fact that Dai was coaching our whole health. I was standing taller. My inner health was improving as much as my outer appearance. The five minutes of still meditation and reflection has often brought me to a place of gratitude. Being still for even five minutes wasn't something I was comfortable with. Now it comes easily and with enjoyment. [Meditation] has transformed from simple deep breathing to reflection." —CHRISTINA

nature, or your challenges, but the main thing is that you don't allow any of it to take a toll on you. Take a deep breath. And take it easy.

Meditation feels great once you learn to relax into it, but at first, it can seem difficult when you try too hard, or are fixated on reaping the benefits NOW! During your early attempts at meditation you might feel frustrated, bored, or even anxious, and that's normal. If this happens to you, simply acknowledge your feelings and then let them go, returning your awareness to your breath, or to your mantra. If your mind wanders aimlessly, accept it and then gently bring your mind back to your meditation.

When you have given your best to your meditation practice, return to your daily activities and notice whether things start to fall into place more effortlessly. Nothing happens overnight, so it pays to be patient! Keep it up and you'll soon feel the difference.

TIME EXPANDS IN THE STILLNESS

As you know, the most common excuse I hear is: *I don't have time*. What if I told you that cultivating a regular meditation practice can actually give you *more* time? How is that possible? Well, when we meditate, we shift in and out of a trance-like state that brings us into contact with a natural inner peace. When we return back to the business of life, we naturally bring this sense of calm into our interactions. (Or, what I like to call the state of pure awesomeness!)

Of course, we can't actually create more hours in the day, unless we happen to be Dr. Who, with access to a time machine! What I'm suggesting is as you start to feel more balanced, calmer and more in-tune with yourself and your surroundings through regular mindfulness practice, you'll develop a greater mental clarity around the things that truly matter most. When I practise mindfulness, even for just five minutes, I find that I'm able to see things much more clearly. I can see what needs my attention right now, and what isn't so important and perhaps doesn't require so much of my time or attention. By following this practice, I free up more time to do things that are truly important to me—the things that put a smile on my face and pep in my step.

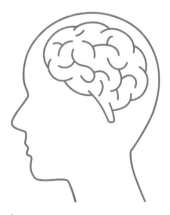

We all get bogged down with the minutia of life. Our calendars are full, but are they full of the things we truly value and need in our life, or are they cluttered with priorities that pull us off our own personal life track? Only you can answer that. Try practising mindful meditation daily and see whether you can accomplish more in less time simply by utilizing your energy more effectively.

YOUR BRAIN ON MEDITATION

Thanks to modern technology, such as magnetic resonance imaging (MRI), scientists are developing a better understanding of what actually takes place in our brains when we meditate.

In a meditative state, the transmission of beta waves in our brain decreases, which means we process information more slowly. The lateral frontal cortex, which is responsible for reasoning, planning, emotions and self-awareness, goes into "sleep mode" during meditation. Meanwhile, the parietal lobe, which detects changes in our environment, slows down during meditation. This is a great thing, especially when trying to maintain a meditative state, as we are able to calm ourselves, relax and ultimately reduce physical and emotional stress.

Meditation can also make your brain bigger! Regular meditative practice has been linked to increased amounts of grey matter in frontal areas of the brain. More grey matter means a greater proportion of positive emotions, more emotional stability, heightened focus and longer attention span.

This does not mean that meditation requires a forced "shutting down" of your brain. Absolutely not! You can't drain your mind of your thoughts—they're part of being human. Numbing out is not our goal in meditation. Instead, we are attempting to reach a natural state of tranquility that already exists in the space *between* our thoughts. Also referred to as "the gap," by Deepak Chopra, this space between thoughts is pure consciousness, silence and peace.

Pick a time of day that works for you. Are you a morning person who would like to begin each day feeling grounded, or would you prefer to meditate to wind down before you go to bed each night? There's no right time except the one that works for you.

It helps to remember that cultivating a meditation practice is a journey, just like developing a physical fitness routine. Mindfulness is like a muscle. If it is not used regularly, it will weaken, but when exercised, it will become a strong and powerful tool.

VICTOR CHAN

Victor Chan is a physicist and writer who studied particle physics at the Enrico Fermi Institute at the University of Chicago. After an introduction through a mutual friend over 40 years ago, Victor Chan has collaborated with His Holiness the Dalai Lama on two books, *The Wisdom of Forgiveness: Intimate Conversations and Travels* and *The Wisdom of Compassion: Stories of Remarkable Encounters and Timeless Insights*. Together, the friends co-founded the Dalai Lama Center for Peace and Education in 2005. In a recent interview, he shared valuable insights about his life, along with his beliefs about mindfulness and meditation.

A number of life experiences fuelled Victor's passion for meditation. Growing up in Hong Kong, he practised tai chi, which he describes as "meditation in motion," and Chinese calligraphy, "another form of meditation." Victor is a long-time adventurer, who spent four years in the 1980s hiking the Tibetan Himalayas; he drew on his experiences there in the 1,100-page *Tibet Handbook: A Pilgrimage Guide*. The 5,486-metre (18,000-foot) passes were incredibly challenging, especially with the added strain of the 23-kg (50-lb) backpack that Victor carried. He applied a special walking meditation during these difficult treks, in which he visualized consciously lowering his metabolic rate. Remarkably, this reduced his sweating significantly.

Later, Victor used aspects of meditation as a university tennis instructor. He taught his beginner students mindfulness techniques that they could apply to their groundstrokes practice. He found that this helped most of his students to pick up the game much faster.

"It's all about using a simple technique to induce focus," he says. "They were able to get into the rhythm early on and were less frustrated by the game."

Today, Victor is a strong believer in using mindfulness in everyday life.

"At the most elementary level, when you want to alleviate some of the stress of life, mindfulness is a good antidote," he suggests. Ultimately, he adds, people who go into a deeper form of meditation have a bigger prize in mind.

"If you pursue it to its logical conclusion, degrees of enlightenment become attainable—it is a concept that's difficult to understand on an intellectual level," explains Victor. "In practical terms, it is possible to live relatively free from stress and free from much of the emotional ups and downs that we experience every day. It's about a happiness that is sustainable and meaningful. It is a worthwhile goal that isn't ephemeral, but very real—but it demands discipline and perseverance."

Striving for "meaningful happiness" sounds awesome to me. How's it sounding to you?

Victor Chan's Meditation Tips:

» As a beginner, **don't be ambitious or try to make it overly complicated**. Five minutes a day is a great place to start, but even two or three minutes is fine.

» **Focus on something simple and basic**. For example, listen to your breath going in and out of your body; you may choose to close your eyes when you do this. Notice the rise and fall of your stomach. Alternatively, you can count from one to 10, then back.

» **Don't divorce meditation from your everyday life**. For example, why not try it when you're chopping vegetables or preparing your meals? Be thoughtful and mindful as you peel and chop a carrot; you can also practise mindfulness as you wash dishes. Perhaps at the start of your meal, try to think about having that mindful approach with each mouthful of food. Or focus on sitting comfortably on a chair.

» **Take it outside!** Try a five-minute walking meditation, in which each step is taken mindfully as your feet lift and lower. Become aware of the feeling under your heels and toes. It may help to do this barefoot.

» **Aim to make it a habit**. Try to sustain a routine for at least a month. This creates a neural groove. Start with a short duration and build up, otherwise you may be overambitious and run the risk of being burnt out.

» **Choose roughly the same time, every day**, which helps to form the habit. You may also try for twice a day.

» Think more about letting mindfulness permeate your everyday life, naturally. **Don't force it**.

» Whenever you can, **try to go with the flow and be in the moment**.

» Acknowledge that meditation is a journey; **don't expect to master it in one session**.

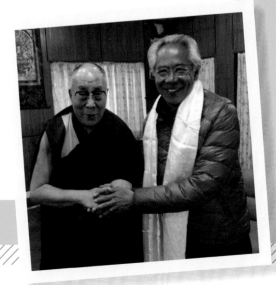

Victor Chan (right) with His Holiness the Dalai Lama.

The overarching aim is to tone your mind and deepen your connection to your spirit. The more challenges life brings your way, the stronger you will emerge.

PERSONAL DEVELOPMENT: PUTTING INSPIRATION INTO PRACTICE

Right after a meditation session, your mind is primed to soak up positive messages and life-enhancing information, making this a great time for personal development activities. This could include reading from an inspiring book, journaling, drawing or writing out your life goals—anything that strengthens your sense of possibility and purpose. You might work on developing a particular talent, boosting your professional potential, or simply enhancing the quality of your relationships through greater self-awareness and better communication skills. Personal development encompasses everything that contributes to the realization of your dreams and aspirations—whatever's most important to YOU!

Have you ever thought about how incredible it is that you've arrived at this exact moment in time, right here and right now? Our lives don't unfold by chance alone. You have made a steady series of choices, right from the time you were first able to conceptualize the ability to choose for yourself, and every one of those choices has led you to this moment in time where you just happen to be reading this passage in this very book.

This type of thinking really opened my mind to bigger questions back in my university days. It put things into a much bigger perspective and made me feel more accountable for the choices I make and the actions I take in my life. And layering this view into my *why*, I find myself wanting to explore even more. To learn more, to live more, to be more—anything that can help me live my purpose and follow my passion.

This is why I feel so strongly about personal development. I think it is essential to constantly push oneself to learn new things, explore new ideas and participate in conversations that expand our understanding of the world and ourselves.

Of course, this is a personal point of view. I've coached many people who feel content with their place in life and don't feel a need to seek out any more answers. Some of them have shared with me that they feel the practice of personal development is an onerous one, and a waste of time. My response to that? *I can't help you.* That's not because I don't care, but because of Newton's First Law:

> An object at rest stays at rest and an object in motion stays in motion with the same speed and in the same direction unless acted upon by an unbalanced force.

At some point in their lives, those individuals' desire to learn, grow and experience life came to a stop. And now they've reached a place that is comfortable and they don't want to rock the boat.

My hope is that you choose to remain in motion. Don't settle for good enough; that is just one step below happiness. As business author Jim Collins says, "Greatness is not a function of circumstance. Greatness, it turns out, is largely a matter of conscious choice, and discipline." Choose greatness! Choose awesomeness! Develop yourself to be the best at whatever passion you have. You have one life to live, so make it the best it can possibly be.

I love this old saying:

> *Be careful with your thoughts, for your thoughts become your words. Be careful with your words, for your words become your actions. Be careful in your actions, for your actions become your habits. Be careful with your habits, for your habits become your character. Be careful of your character, for your character becomes your destiny.*
> —Frank Outlaw, late president of Bi-Lo

So, how are you thinking, speaking and acting? What do you choose to listen to, read and watch, each and every day? Feed your mind, and your life will change. Now, go forth and plant seeds of awesomeness in your mind's garden!

"At the beginning, I was super leery of joining the Whole Life Fitness Power 30. I thought I would give up quickly and not complete the workout of the day. Well, I'm happy to report, I'm completing each day to the best of my ability. I've positively changed in so many ways; I feel stronger, healthier and more alert—and I'm getting better at meditation." —FEATHER

CHECK FOOD LABELS

LIVE LIFE DELICIOUS

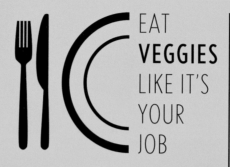

EAT **VEGGIES** LIKE IT'S YOUR JOB

Have protein first thing in the morning

GO MEATLESS

1 MEAL {OR} DAY / PER WEEK

Find healthy foods that you to eat

WEIGHT LOSS IS A SIDE EFFECT OF **HEALTH**

FORGET **CALORIE-COUNTING**

EAT A **BALANCED** DIET

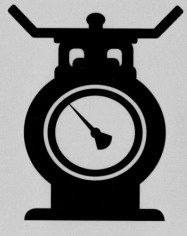

FOLLOW THE 10% RULE

=

90% HEALTHY

+

10% ON THE SWEET SIDE

Think moderation

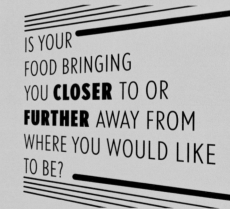

IS YOUR FOOD BRINGING YOU **CLOSER** TO OR **FURTHER** AWAY FROM WHERE YOU WOULD LIKE TO BE?

AN EXTRA **150** CALORIES PER DAY OVER WHAT OUR BODY NEEDS

=

AN EXTRA **15** LBS OF WEIGHT GAIN PER YEAR.

EAT SMART

MOST OF US HAVE STRUGGLED with food at some point in our lives. And it's not hard to see why—understanding good nutrition can be confusing. Every day we are bombarded with the latest food fads, including new-fangled celebrity diets, and what so-called food experts tell us we should never put in our shopping cart again.

I am intimately aware of the challenges of healthy eating. Before digging into some simple nutritional guidelines, I'd like to share some more about my previous relationship with food.

During my teens, when I decided to lose weight and get healthy, I had a strict list of 10 "safe" foods that I allowed myself to eat: cottage cheese, yogurt, chicken, tuna, rice, sweet potatoes or yams, almonds, salad greens, apples and cantaloupes. I never deviated from it. I successfully worked my way out of obesity, but my limited diet was not sustainable. My diet became something that controlled me, rather than something that I controlled, and it wore me down emotionally and mentally.

The true meaning of the word *diet* is not "restrictive eating plan," but quite simply, "the foods we eat." Our diet is meant to provide us with the fuel we need to nourish ourselves; it includes the vitamins, minerals and nutrients we need for our bodies and minds.

Within a few years, I tired of harsh restrictive eating, and of constantly telling myself *no*. *No* to the piece of cake at a friend's birthday party, *no* to cream in my coffee, *no* to juice, *no* to fruits I thought contained too much natural sugar, *no* to muffins and other baked goods, and *no* to new food experiences because I didn't feel they would fit my lifestyle. In hindsight, I missed out on a lot of great flavours and cultural experiences because of my rigid outlook, and my warped understanding of the word *diet*.

> "Dai has inspired me in so many ways. He's always so full of energy, is encouraging, and in high spirits. He's a wonderful parent, coach and human being. He makes workouts fun and they're always different. He has always been there for me with any questions or concerns, and never gave up on me when I was feeling low. He has made me more conscious about what I eat, my water intake, and how important it is to be a better, healthier me. He literally changed my life."—MEAGAN

WHAT'S YOUR EATING STYLE?

How would you describe your eating style? Are you a person who scarfs down or gobbles up your food? If so, it's time to change. Become someone who savours every morsel, and chews every mouthful.

Food is a significant part of our cultural development. Along with death and taxes, the need to eat is one of the great constants in life. Why not explore the health benefits of all foods, and develop a positive relationship with the way we nourish our communities and ourselves?

As my take on food has evolved over the years, one hand-on-heart mantra has emerged: *Realistic, doable, practical, liveable.* The trouble with an overly restrictive eating plan is that it just won't last, because it will become so tiresome! Remember, if you aren't having fun with something, it will start to feel like work rather than a lifestyle choice, and it will eventually grind to a halt.

Every one of the food choices we make throughout the day will either help or hinder us from achieving our health goals. These goals ultimately come down to each of us as individuals. One of my main motivators to stay on a healthy eating path is to envision what my life might be like in 10, 20 or 30 years' time. With each food-related decision I make, I fast-forward into the future and pose the question: *Are these mouthfuls bringing me closer to where I would like to be, or further away?*

Personally, I'm inspired to eat my way towards a picture of health expressed in Michelangelo's *David*. This sculpture represents one of my physical ideals, so I proudly keep pictures of it on my vision boards. (A *vision board* is a tool that includes inspirational quotes and images to help a person visualize desired future outcomes as a reminder of what's possible.) *David* looks athletic, healthy and has great proportions, but he's not a muscle-bound freak.

So ask yourself how you want to look in 20 years. If your honest truth is your current diet is dragging you further away from your ideal future, then the choice in front of you should be fairly clear.

> " Let food be thy medicine, thy medicine shall be thy food."
>
> —HIPPOCRATES

I understand that occasionally we slip up, and I think that's okay, too. Balance is about owning our decisions, being conscious of our choices, being proud of our eating habits and not stressing! *Diet* may be a four-letter word, but so is *love*, so move forward with love for your food, and for yourself!

I do my best to eat balanced meals every day. As a family, the majority of the time we aim to consume a Paleolithic diet, sometimes known as the *caveman diet*, which puts the emphasis on whole foods: fruits and vegetables, grass-fed beef, poultry

> "Healthy eating is not something you do for a while when you're trying to improve your fitness. It's a change for the better that becomes a way of life."

and fish, as well as nuts and good fats. Foods that are excluded include sugar, dairy products, salt, processed oils and gluten-rich grains. We eat organic foods as much as possible. As my wife Christie often says, "Beige is bad, greens are good!" which is a playful guideline to bear in mind when you sit down to eat. That's not to say you can never eat a bagel or pasta, but defaulting to them just because they are convenient or because you find yourself craving them isn't the greatest way to nourish yourself. Honestly, our family feels physically and mentally better for these so-called "restrictions." Although, we never view them as restrictions—to us they are enhancements, or better yet, our lifestyle.

One sure-fire tip for becoming more conscious of your food is to take a picture of everything you are about to put in your mouth over a single day, a 72-hour period, or perhaps a week. This will help you to see what, when and how much you're eating and drinking. A number of fitness professionals recommend weighing every morsel of food and drink that enters your body, or to document everything you eat in a journal. I don't know how well this works, but I do know that most of us have smartphones with us all of the time, so it's easy to take a quick picture of anything you're about to consume. After a few days, you'll get a good sense of where you are with your current eating habits. This exercise in documenting your nutrition can be an eye-opening experience.

Good nutrition not only keeps you alive, but it also lifts your energy levels, boosts your mood, keeps your skin and hair looking good and helps you to maintain a healthy weight. Undeniably, good nutrition is the obvious partner of exercise in health and fitness success.

Healthy eating is not something you do for a while when you're trying to improve your fitness. Don't think of it as temporary, or something that you'll abandon once you reach your goal weight (if you have one). Healthy eating is a change for the better that becomes a new way of life.

KATHY SMART'S NUTRITION TIPS

Kathy Smart is one of the most infectiously enthusiastic food experts I've ever met. A holistic chef, nutritionist, host of her own TV show, *Live The Smart Way*, and author of *Live the Smart Way: Gluten-Free & Wheat-Free Cookbook*, Kathy is a strong advocate of the food-as-a-lifestyle philosophy. For this book, I interviewed her to get her best nutrition tips.

To help people return to—or find for the first time—that "feel-good state," Kathy encourages people to integrate a healthier nutritional plan into their lifestyle. She sets people up for success by establishing basic nutritional guidelines on which types of food—and which combinations—are best on your plate. The message is clear: Change how you eat, and you will change how you feel. And who doesn't want to feel great?

Kathy emphasizes the importance of balance with most of the meals we eat, including:

- **A muscle-building protein hit:** This might be in the form of fish, such as halibut or salmon; meats, such as chicken, lamb and beef; dairy; or eggs. Vegans can choose plant-based proteins, such as tempeh, or a wide range of nuts and legumes.
- **Fibre-rich, complex carbohydrates:** That applies to gluten-free whole grains, such as quinoa and corn, as well as other whole grains, such as barley. She recommends steering away from traditional forms of fibre, such as bran-rich bread, which is often over-processed. Instead, think outside of the box. Did you know, for example, that coconut flour has 58 per cent fibre, compared to wheat bran, which contains only 27 per cent? Also, consider starchy, fibre-rich vegetables such as Swiss chard, yams, peas or broccoli.
- **Low-GI vegetables:** These include asparagus, bell peppers, cabbage, celery, collard greens, cucumbers, fennel bulbs, kale, romaine lettuce, and other high-fibre, low starch, low-sugar veggies.
- **Healthy fats:** These might be found in your proteins, or you might think of serving a small portion of unsaturated fats on their own. For example, almonds contain monounsaturated fats, which help to reduce cholesterol levels.

ESTIMATED CALORIE NEEDS PER DAY
BY AGE, GENDER AND PHYSICAL ACTIVITY LEVEL*

GENDER	AGE (YEARS)	PHYSICAL ACTIVITY LEVEL**		
		SEDENTARY	MODERATELY ACTIVE	ACTIVE
Child (female and male)	2-3	1,000-1,200***	1,000-1,400***	1,000-1,400***
Female****	4-8	1,200-1,400	1,400-1,600	1,400-1,800
	9-13	1,400-1,600	1,600-2,000	1,800-2,200
	14-18	1,800	2,000	2,400
	19-30	1,800-2,000	2,000-2,200	2,400
	31-50	1,800	2,000	2,200
	51+	1,600	1,800	2,000-2,200
Male	4-8	1,200-1,400	1,400-1,600	1,600-2,000
	9-13	1,600-2,000	1,800-2,200	2,000-2,600
	14-18	2,000-2,400	2,400-2,800	2,800-3,200
	19-30	2,400-2,600	2,600-2,800	3,000
	31-50	2,200-2,400	2,400-2,600	2,800-3,000
	51+	2,000-2,200	2,200-2,400	2,400-2,800

HEALTH.GOV DIETARY GUIDELINES, 2010

Note: Estimated amounts of calories needed to maintain calorie balance for various gender and age groups at three different levels of physical activity. The estimates are rounded to the nearest 200 calories. An individual's calorie needs may be higher or lower than these average estimates.

* Based on Estimated Energy Requirements (EER) equations, using reference heights (average) and reference weights (healthy) for each age/gender group. For children and adolescents, reference height and weight vary. For adults, the reference man is 178 cm (5 ft 10 in) tall and weighs 70 kg (154 lbs). The reference woman is 163 cm (5 ft 4 in) tall and weighs 57 kg (126 lbs). EER equations are from the Institute of Medicine. Dietary Reference Intakes for Energy, Carbohydrate, Fibre, Fat, Fatty Acids, Cholesterol, Protein and Amino Acids. Washington (DC): The National Academies Press; 2002.

** Sedentary means a lifestyle that includes only the light physical activity associated with typical day-to-day life. Moderately active means a lifestyle that includes physical activity equivalent to walking about 2.4 to 4.8 km (1.5 to 3 mi) per day at 4.8 to 6.4 kph (3 to 4 mph), in addition to the light physical activity associated with typical day-to-day life. Active means a lifestyle that includes physical activity equivalent to walking more than 4.8 km (3 mi) per day at 4.8 to 6.4 kph (3 to 4 mph), in addition to the light physical activity associated with typical day-to-day life.

*** The calorie ranges shown are to accommodate needs of different ages within the group. For children and adolescents, more calories are needed at older ages. For adults, fewer calories are needed at older ages.

**** Estimates for females do not include women who are pregnant or breastfeeding.

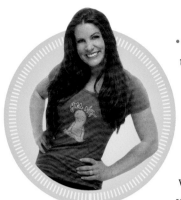

- **Fruit:** From bananas to oranges, have a small portion on the side of each meal.

Once you've worked out your food groups and you know how to put together a balanced, nutritious meal, here's the crunch question: *How much can you eat?*

Kathy explains that portion size depends on who you are, that is, whether you are male or female, your age and activity levels, your height and your size. What's right for you may not be right for your best friend, so remember that guidelines are based on general principles, and it's up to each of us to work out how our bodies respond. Women usually require fewer calories than men, but an extremely active woman may require more than an inactive man.

"Basically, everyone is different, so these recommendations may not be entirely right for you," Kathy explains.

As a simple guideline, it's useful to aim to fill half of your plate with vegetables and the other half with equal portions of protein and complex carbohydrates.

"Thinking along these balanced lines at every meal or snack covers a lot of your nutritional bases," she says.

But what do these figures actually look like at your meal times? We all know that plate—and therefore portion—sizes can differ, so Kathy recommends that people refer to their hand to work out how much food they should be consuming. After all, everyone's hand size is proportional to their body size, and no matter where you are (at a party, work function, or eating in a restaurant), you always have your hand with you! With no pun intended, it's a "handy" guide to getting your portions right.

"It keeps it really simple," says Kathy. "I'm not a big fan of people weighing and measuring their food, because I think that food should be something that's a joy and not restrictive like a science experiment." So put away those kitchen scales, right now!

When we don't immediately need the fuel (glucose) in the food we're eating, the body stores it as glycogen in the liver and skeletal muscles. If our glycogen capacity is full, that glucose is stored as fat. When we exercise, this glycogen is depleted from the muscles. Immediately after exercising, we're in what Kathy calls a "golden hour" for building muscle tissue. That means that eating a nutritionally balanced snack within an hour of intense activity helps to refuel your muscles right when they need it most. Ideally, this should be a snack-size portion of the perfect combination of

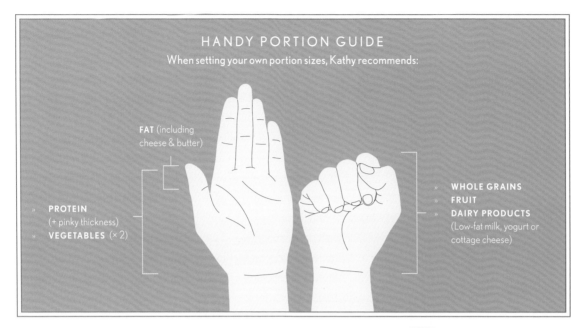

HANDY PORTION GUIDE

When setting your own portion sizes, Kathy recommends:

FAT (including cheese & butter)

» **PROTEIN** (+ pinky thickness)
» **VEGETABLES** (× 2)

» **WHOLE GRAINS**
» **FRUIT**
» **DAIRY PRODUCTS** (Low-fat milk, yogurt or cottage cheese)

protein, complex carbohydrate and fat. For a well-balanced snack that's great on-the-go, try Kathy's High Energy Maca Balls, made from oats, cinnamon, pumpkin seeds, flax seeds, raisins and the superfood maca—a Peruvian root revered by generations as an energy enhancer and mood stabilizer, which can be found in powder form in many health food stores.

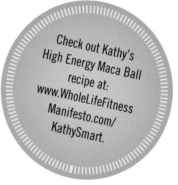

Check out Kathy's High Energy Maca Ball recipe at: www.WholeLifeFitnessManifesto.com/KathySmart.

A NEW FOOD ATTITUDE

Having established which foods to aim for and how much, is the idea of eating well starting to feel like a chore? Well, those days are over. Kathy is passionate about giving healthy food a creative makeover. She's leading a nutritional movement and ensuring it's uncomplicated, convenient and downright yummy.

And she's had some pretty tough critics to satisfy over nearly two decades in the business. When her cookbook received the seal of approval from *Le Cordon Bleu*, the renowned culinary school, Kathy felt she had cleared a big hurdle.

"If people who were used to fine, rich food ate and liked my recipes, and didn't know it was healthy, then my job was done."

TRY THESE RECIPES! Get these recipes and more from www.WholeLifeFitness Manifesto.com /KathySmart.

Just as I encourage people to find an exercise they love to do, Kathy stresses that we need to find healthy foods that we love to eat—and to make it delicious. It's *that* simple.

"I think there is a preconceived notion of people thinking that healthy food is gross," Kathy explains. So she makes sure she gives people healthy choices that taste good to them specifically. "Honour their palate. So if they have a more savoury palate, obviously give them more savoury, or if it's more sweet, then give them healthier sweet choices, because as humans we're always going to gravitate to things we like."

So, what's your palate like? Are you drawn to mixed greens with dried cherries and goat cheese, spicy chicken with creamy peanut sauce, or Mediterranean-style salmon? Perhaps you'd enjoy desserts such as Kathy's healthier versions of pecan maple date scones, double fudge brownies or high-protein tempeh chocolate cake? (See? Repeat after me: *Wholesome diets don't need to be boring!*) Whatever your preference, it's worth evoking the old adage, *Everything in moderation*, to ensure you have a balanced diet, which runs from breakfast through to your evening meal.

Another of Kathy's top tips is to always have protein within an hour of waking up. For anyone who suffers from a mid-morning slump or afternoon cravings, this advice is significant. If you're having cravings, or even late-night binges, look back at your breakfast. This relates to the GI rating of the foods you eat.

"When you have protein first thing in the morning, it helps to stabilize your blood sugar for the whole day," she explains. "This will have a domino effect, and will set you up to succeed." To make this success truly sustainable and enjoyable, pick a high-protein or low-GI food that you really like, she advises, such as steel-cut oats, smoked salmon, or zesty omelettes. "Going for a couple of pieces of toast and orange juice at breakfast will spike your blood sugar, and what goes up must come down," Kathy explains. "When it comes down, you start to crave sugar and carbohydrates and so you're up and down all day, and therefore you get moody."

Understanding how food affects our moods is crucial. We all notice if our kids are bouncing off the wall after eating cake or candy. The immediate effects of different foods are not necessarily so obvious in adults, so I encourage my clients to look through the pictures of the food they took that day and figure out which foods are or aren't working for them, based on how they feel an hour after eating them.

Notice your physiological reactions after eating: Are you feeling satisfied and light, are you still hungry, or are you feeling bloated and heavy? Also notice how you feel emotionally and energetically: Are you upbeat and raring to go, or sluggish and low? These are all descriptors you can replay in your mind next time you consider eating a piece of sugary chocolate cake, a slice of triple-cheese pizza, or a mountain of heavily buttered toast.

Our eating and exercise habits constantly return us to the fact that we are making choices that affect our long-term well-being throughout the day, every day. By taking note of our experiences and our responses to them, we will soon naturally begin to see what the right choices are for *us*.

"You need to know how you feel after certain foods, and certain amounts of food, to really start working out what is correct for you," Kathy says. "If you have a healthy relationship with your body—how it looks, how it feels, how it moves—you'll soon discover that it's paramount to have a healthy relationship with food."

The meaning that we give food and the way in which we connect with it play a huge part in our overall health, beyond the battle of the bulge.

"It's so important to make those healthy choices because you want to feel amazing and awesome—not just because you're going to lose weight," Kathy says. "Weight loss is a side effect of health. You don't lose weight and then become healthy. There are a lot of skinny-fat unhealthy people out there. You can lose weight by smoking cigarettes and drinking diet cola!" Clearly, not a healthy way to live.

Another suggestion for working toward a great relationship with healthy food comes from Don Warren, Kathy's long-time naturopathic doctor. Kathy cites this as one of the most lingering nuggets of nutritional advice she's heard because it evokes such a powerful visual.

KATHY SMART'S HEALTHY HITS

» **Hemp seeds:** Their essential fatty acids help to reduce inflammation and boost your skin, nails and hair.
» **Apple cider vinegar:** Helps with weight loss (take a spoonful before eating).
» **Cinnamon:** Just half a teaspoon helps reduce cholesterol.
» **Eggs:** For naturally occurring vitamin D.
» **Asparagus:** Helps cleanse the kidneys and prevents the formation of kidney stones.
» **Black onion seeds:** To help detoxify the liver and reduce inflammation.

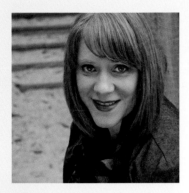

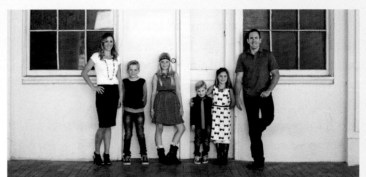

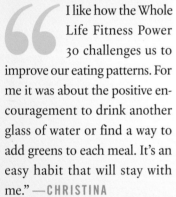

> I like how the Whole Life Fitness Power 30 challenges us to improve our eating patterns. For me it was about the positive encouragement to drink another glass of water or find a way to add greens to each meal. It's an easy habit that will stay with me." —CHRISTINA

> I met Dai at a relatively random business dinner in Las Vegas. Over the course of several non-alcoholic beverages Dai taught me about CrossFit and how he encouraged people to eat well and be active. I could sense right away that he had a passion for helping people achieve their fitness goals. When I got home I looked up the local CrossFit gym and committed to getting back into shape. Now I am a partner in several gyms and am healthier in my 30s than I was in my 20s. It's amazing what a little spark can do when it fuels somebody's desire to change their life. Thank you for being the spark, Dai!" —TYLER

"He told me to eat vegetables like it's my job to eat as many vegetables as I can," she says, adding that research is continually stressing their role in helping to fight cancer and heart disease, among other health complaints. "Because they fill you up with all that nutrition and goodness, you won't even want other food or crave sugar. This will change how anyone eats."

Kathy uses two glass containers to portion out about 960 mL (four cups) of vegetables to be eaten each day. If she's on the run, she takes her veggies along for the ride in plastic baggies. Et voila…goodbye sugar cravings, hello satisfying nutrition. My equivalent is having what I like to call a BAHG (big-ass healthy green) salad every day!

We all know there can be days when it seems you're too busy to even chop vegetables, but Kathy has an answer for that, too.

"If it feels like an overwhelming task, I will buy a vegetable tray."

If you eat enough vegetables, Kathy swears you won't crave sugar. If, however, you find that you still do, there are other factors you can look at beyond your breakfast and your vegetable intake. For example, how much restful sleep are you getting at night? Are you going to bed immediately after an evening of watching TV or being on the computer—or, worse, with the blue light of your smartphone or tablet near you?

"I can tell people to eat baby carrots instead of ice cream, but if they are actually craving sugar because their body hasn't slept and recuperated, that carrot thing ain't going to work," Kathy says. "That's about their body needing an extra hit."

Consider, then, whether you are setting yourself up for a successful, undisturbed night's rest. Could you go to bed earlier, or turn off the electronics at winding-down time? Your energy levels will thank you.

There are a lot of rules making the rounds about eating in the evening, such as *no food past 7 p.m.*, but Kathy doesn't go for arbitrary cut-off times. Instead, she suggests that you avoid eating food within three hours of your bedtime, whatever time that may be.

"It's a tough one because so many people work shift work, such as nurses, doctors, journalists and firefighters, so having a set time doesn't always apply," she says. "This is an easier guide that can accommodate everybody."

HYDRATION

Keeping well hydrated is vital to fighting fatigue, lifting our spirits and making us perform and feel better. This is as important when we're working out as it is to when we're at home and at work. After all, as Kathy Smart reminds us, precious water makes up two-thirds of our body weight. Water can also help to curb hunger pangs. Try drinking a glass of water the next time you think you're hungry and see if you still feel ravenous afterwards. Kathy also has some great recipes for healthy vitamin waters, with flavours ranging from sage to pineapple.

NO NAME-CALLING!

It may be double-cooked French fries for one person, or an ice-cream sundae with extra whipped cream and chocolate sprinkles for another. Who isn't tempted by their favourite indulgent treat once in a while?

Before we go any further, I want to veer into the hot debate over labelling food as either "bad" or "good," and "right" or "wrong." Personally, I believe in *reading* food labels, not *labelling* food! Okay, Christie and I do have fun with our "beige is bad, green is good" mantra, but really, we're not demonizing beige foods.

Taking a moral stand against particular foods will not help you to develop a positive relationship with your body and the food that goes into it. I encourage all of my clients to take a non-judgmental approach to food. Rather than strict calorie counting and chastising yourself when you go over your set limit, try to think of food as a nourishing and enjoyable support system for your whole life. If you can make your food routine fun, too, you're more likely to stick with it.

Each of us is fully empowered to make our own decisions, as we're the ones who have to live with the repercussions of those decisions. It's so important to recognize that you're in the driver's seat of your own decisions, not bound by someone else's "rules."

How do you perceive the foods you choose to eat? Do you feel guilty about certain foods? Why is that? If these questions create strong emotions, it may be time to shift your perspective.

Sometimes, cultural norms dictate our perceptions of particular foods. For example, did you know that in France, chocolate cake is associated with fun, revelry, and celebration? It is a special dessert with a positive meaning. In North America, however, chocolate cake is often seen as a "guilty pleasure." Knowing that these labels and associations aren't set in stone can give you the freedom to re-examine your own assumptions about food.

So, be it resolved: We're not going to demonize the food we eat. But how do we resist the constant temptation of junk food and sweets? Can we use these treats as a way to occasionally motivate ourselves?

I'll be honest: There are nights when I want a piece of cheesecake, and nothing is going to stop me from having it. I'm a big believer in the benefits of having a "cheat meal," or at least taking a break from my traditional way of eating. Pick one day each week and call it your "free meal" day, and on that day, enjoy one meal that falls outside of your normal everyday lifestyle. On my "free day" I like to enjoy a few slices of pizza followed by a big bowl of ice cream! What's your ideal "free meal" of choice? Tweet me! During the rest of the week, knowing that your free meal is coming can help you behave on the other days.

This concept is one that Kathy Smart backs wholeheartedly. Whatever your indulgence, Kathy advises to, "Make it amazing, and don't cheap out on it. If you have some French fries on a Friday cheat night, it's not going to be the end of the world. Have a couple of bites, enjoy it, make it the most decadent thing, and then you will find you won't want it anymore."

DINING OUT TIPS

» Stay away from dressings (they often are loaded with sugar). Ask for lemon wedges, balsamic vinegar or apple cider vinegar.

» Ask for no seasoning or light seasoning on meats. There's a reason why restaurant food tastes so flavourful!

» Ask for your veggies to be steamed. Otherwise, you might be served flash-fried veggies.

» Choose salad (remember the dressing trick though!) over french fries. This might be hard at first, but you know you'll feel better after!

» Club soda with a lime wedge is always a good beverage choice and refills are often free!

You may even choose to satisfy your craving with a version of your favourite treat made with whole sweeteners, such as maple syrup, honey, agave nectar or brown rice syrup, rather than refined sugar, corn syrup, glucose or sucrose. But my feeling is that if you really want the full fat, full sugar, full cream versions of your lust-have foods, just own the decision to eat them and enjoy them.

These occasional "cheat" moments are not meant to encourage binge eating. Kathy urges us to think in terms of moderation. Kathy recommends what she calls the "10 per cent rule." This means that if 90 per cent of your diet is clean and healthy, you can indulge in treats for the other 10 per cent. She's also a big fan of dark chocolate, which she describes as a "hit of happiness" that also happens to have appetite-suppressing properties. Now that's a tasty thought!

"Everything comes down to balance," Kathy stresses. "Food is to be enjoyed. One of the psychological benefits of eating food you love is that the feel-good chemicals released in the brain outweigh some of the detrimental effects of, say, a little cheesecake."

Now that sounds good. Or, to quote her wonderful catchphrase, healthy eating is all about us trying to "live life delicious."

CHEAP AND CHEERFUL

Kathy Smart's cheap and cheerful ways to eat healthy:

» Go meatless for one meal or day per week. Instead, use beans—take your pick from protein-filled adzuki to black beans, from garbanzo to kidney.

» Peel and freeze bananas, then use them to make banana bread or add them to smoothies.

» Don't be afraid to check out the reduced section in the grocery store for vegetables. When you get them home, chop and freeze them as soon as possible to preserve them at their freshest.

» Ask and receive: Contact companies of healthy products that you love or want to try. They may send out free samples or coupons. "If you love their product, you are going to tell everyone," Kathy says, "and the best advertisement is word of mouth."

IT'S TIME TO GET STARTED!

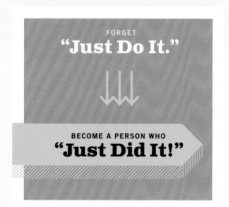

FORGET
"Just Do It."

BECOME A PERSON WHO
"Just Did It!"

HERE'S WHERE THE *Whole Life Fitness Manifesto* is going to really move you. We've reasoned through it all. You've identified and overcome the barriers that once stopped you from making a change for the better in your life. You've identified your *why*. Exterminated the externalizers. And, you've thought realistically about your time constraints, figuring out how you can allot health and fitness into your busy schedule.

It's time to forget being a "Just Do It" person, and shoot for being somebody who "Just Did It!"

But first, a word about the most important piece of exercise equipment out there...

JUST BUY THE SHOES!

In nearly two decades of selling fitness equipment, I saw a lot of people stress out about their gear. I would hear the same concerns and questions again and again: "What's the best piece of equipment for fat-burning?" "Is this like the thing I saw on TV that will get me fit and skinny in only six minutes a day?" "What's the single best piece of equipment for a full-body workout?" "Which is best: treadmill, elliptical machine, exercise bike or rowing machine?"

I saw a lot of stereotypes when couples came into the store together. The men often wanted a home gym filled with weights, while the women wanted cardio, cardio, cardio. Many women worried that lifting weights would cause them to bulk up. (Note to female readers: Using weights will NOT cause you to bulk up!)

Do you see what's going on here? Lots of misinformation, paired with a deep desire to find a fast and reliable solution. I hate to be the bearer of bad news, but there's no magic pill, no one piece of equipment that will do it all for you.

Let's be honest. The fitness equipment industry has some nasty clichés and stereotypes associated with it. Visit a garage sale or check out your local Craigslist for-sale listings and you'll see a long list of barely-used gym equipment, purchased with the best of intentions, but unwanted nonetheless. Why is this?

There are a number of common culprits, such as buying the wrong piece of equipment for your personal preferences. (If you don't like the modality of riding a bike, for example, why would you subject yourself to doing it every day?) Sometimes just the placement of the equipment is to blame. For instance, putting your new gym equipment in your basement—when it's the last place in your house you'd ever want to spend time—isn't the best way to motivate yourself to use it. And then there's my personal favourite: "My doctor told me to buy it." Seriously. I've heard this more often than you would think.

Don't get me wrong; I think gym equipment is amazing! I love using different types of equipment, but they don't make or break a workout for me. They are tools I can choose to leverage when I have access to them.

Think of exercise equipment as a vacuum or dishwasher. These are fantastic appliances that help us complete housework more efficiently, but what did we do before we had them? We washed dishes by hand and we swept our floors with a broom. So think of fitness equipment as amazing tools (or, as I say, toys) that can add diversity to your workouts, but don't let a lack of equipment or gym access limit your exercise and fitness.

Listening to the tortured debates in the store, I really wanted to tell many customers to *just buy the shoes!* As wonderful as gym equipment can be, it's not going to make you move in the first place; that has to come from you. Simply buying the sneakers (or not) underscores the basic premise of fitness: Getting fit comes from your own motivation to move and change your life.

Be clear and realistic about your goals

A RECIPE FOR FITNESS SUCCESS

Aim to MOVE your body with PURPOSE each day.

BEGIN WITH THE EXERCISES YOU ENJOY AND BRING A SMILE TO YOUR FACE

STAY STRONG AND FOCUSED

MAKE #JUSTDIDIT ONE OF YOUR DAILY MANTRAS

KEEP SQUATTING

WE ALL WANT TO GET IN AND OUT OF A CHAIR, RIGHT?

Find an ACCOUNT-A-BUDDY —someone to hold you accountable— like your FAMILY, FRIENDS and ONLINE COMMUNITY.

Your range of motion may be limited in the beginning, but focus on proper form and you will get better!

MOST OF ALL, REMEMBER WHY YOU'RE DOING IT

THE FIRST STEP IN THE Whole Life Fitness Power 30 is to become familiar with the basic exercise moves—there are 34 in total. Each movement is broken down from a start position to an end position. We've offered some variations to try on some of the movements, because everyone starts the program with a different level of fitness. Don't fret if you have to use the variations at first—that's why we've provided them. It's important to remember that there's no judgment here. Just do each movement to the best of your ability, and keep moving.

Remember to be mindful of your own limits, not your friend's. Work within your range of motion and at an intensity that works for you. You may feel a little discomfort at times, but you should not feel any pain (Remember: *No pain, no pain!*). Always consult a physician before starting any new exercise program.

And try to be patient with yourself. Nothing happens overnight. The Whole Life Fitness Power 30 is not an instant fix; it's a sustainable, practical, doable solution toward a more fit and healthy life. It works bit-by-bit, day-by-day, and inch-by-inch. If we keep reinforcing these new positive habits, the big payoff is sure to come.

PLEASE NOTE: Always consult your physician before beginning any exercise program.

ICON GUIDE

♡ CARDIO   ◉ FEXIBILITY

⬆ CORE   ⚡ STRENGTH

" The person who says it cannot be done should not interrupt the person who is doing it"

—CHINESE PROVERB

NEUTRAL STANCE

LANDING POSITION

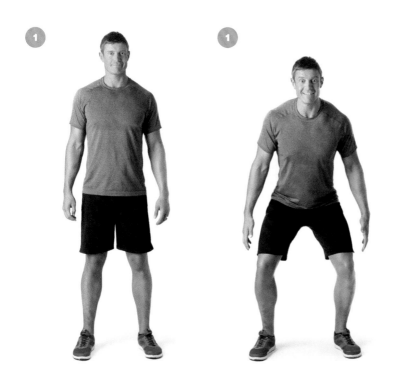

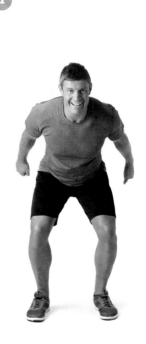

Stand with your feet hip-width apart, core tight, with a proud (lifted) chest. Feel your centre of gravity running down from your upper body into your feet.

Allow your hips, knees and ankles to absorb the impact when you land. Many will find that a natural landing stance is with the knees slightly bent, and the feet a little wider than hip-width apart.

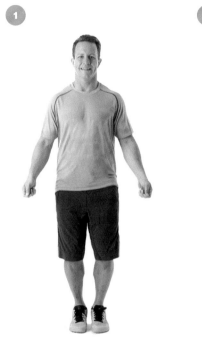

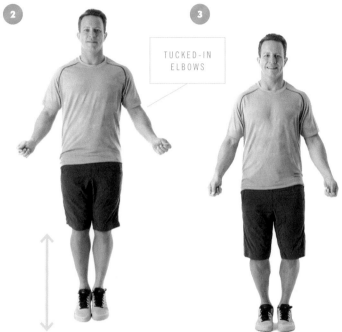

TUCKED-IN ELBOWS

1 Stand with your feet together. Be light on the balls of your feet (lift your heels up and down to feel it).

2 Jump slightly as you rotate your wrists as if you were twirling a skipping rope.

3 Allow your hips, knees and ankles to absorb the impact when you land.

KEY POINTS

» Keep your core engaged, posture upright while you bounce up and down on both feet simultaneously.

» Keep your elbows tucked into your sides and your hands at hip level.

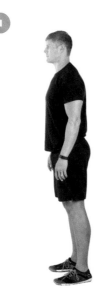

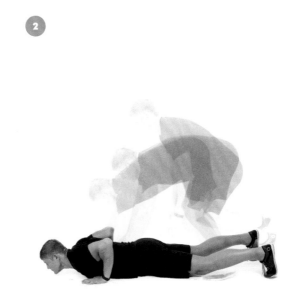

1 Start in neutral stance.

2 Drop your body into a push-up—chest to the ground, legs outstretched, on your toes.

3 Extend your arms as if doing a push-up, then bring your feet back up toward your hands.

4 Come up to standing and do a small jump, extending the hips at the top.

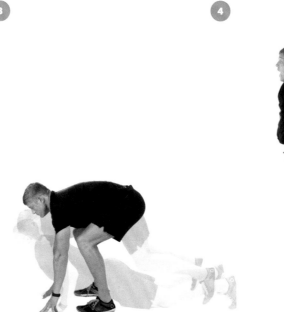

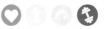

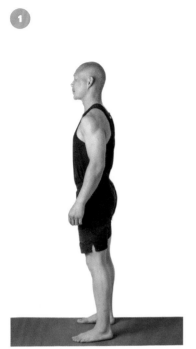

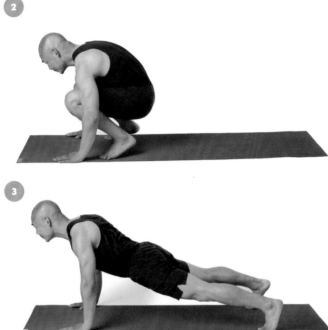

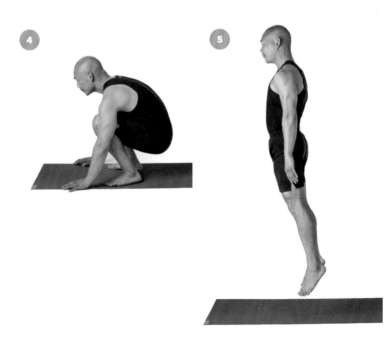

1 Start in neutral stance.

2 Squat down, bringing hands to the ground in front of you.

3 Kick feet out into a plank position with legs in a "V" position.

4 Jump your feet back in toward the hands.

5 Stand up and do a slight jump extending the hips at the top, arms by your side.

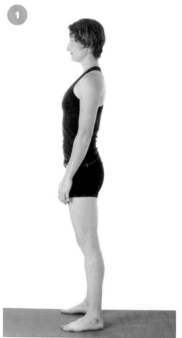

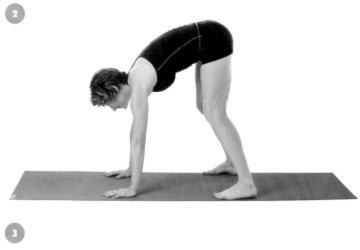

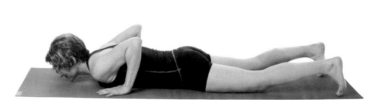

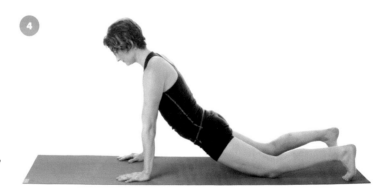

1 Neutral stance.

2 Bend your knees and bring your hands to the floor.

3 Walk hands out until you are flat on the floor with hands tucked under your shoulders, palms pressed into the floor.

4 Press up from the floor raising your upper body until your arms are straight.

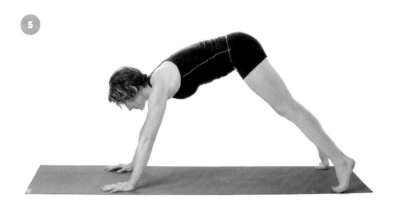

5 Lift hips up into the air, creating an inverted "V".

6 Walk hands back towards your feet until you are in a squat position.

7 Jump into the air while fully straightening your body. Feet only need to leave the ground slightly.

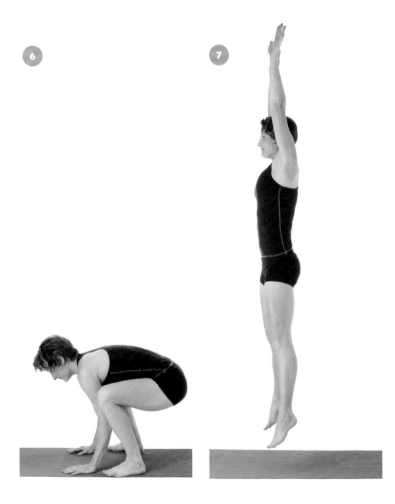

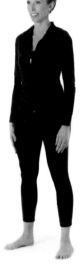
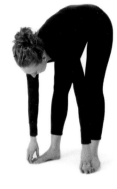
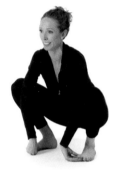
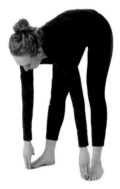

1 Start in neutral stance.

2 Bend forward from the waist, keeping legs and back straight. Aim to touch your toes (if you can't touch, don't stress, go to where you are comfortable.)

3 While holding onto your toes, pull hips down into a squat position. Note that weight should be on your heels, not toes. Maintain a proud chest, use your arms to help press knees outward.

4 While keeping your grip on your toes, lift your hips into the air until legs are straightened.

5 Walk your hands out (5a) along the floor until you are lying face down (5b). Press hands firmly into the floor, while keeping your elbows tucked in alongside your rib cage.

6 Engage your abs by tilting your pelvis forward, and draw your belly button in toward your spine. Push your upper body off the floor and straighten your arms as much as it is comfortable. Aim to keep a neutral neck, with your legs and feet planted firmly on the floor. Pause for a 2 second count.

7 Release tension in your body by lowering the upper body back down towards the floor, while raising your hips up into the air, entering into an inverted "V" position.

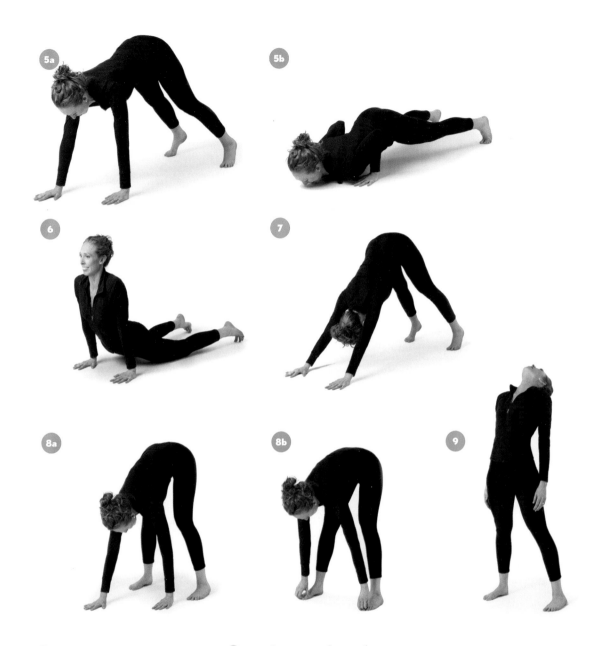

8 Walk hands back towards your feet (8a) until they touch your toes (or back into a position that you are comfortable in) (8b).

9 Stand up, completing the movement with a light backbend, while pressing your hips slightly forward to release your hip flexors.

1 Lie flat on your back,
knees bent, feet placed
hip-width apart below your
bottom. Place hands lightly
against knees.

2 Curl up, slowly lifting your
neck and shoulder blades
off the mat, followed by
the rest of your back.
Imagine your midsection is
a sponge that you're wring-
ing out as you contract your
abdominal muscles.

3 Pause for a second, then
return your mid-back, and
then your shoulders back
down to the mat.

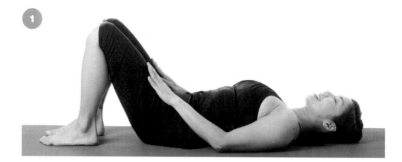

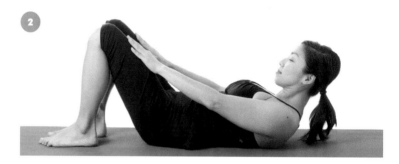

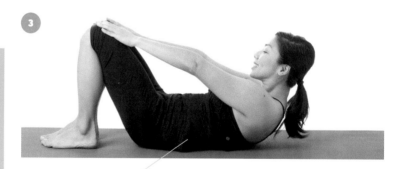

KEY POINTS

» Breathe out as you
elevate, breathe in as you
lower down.
» Slow, controlled movements,
keeping tension in
the midsection.

PUSH LOWER BACK TO
GROUND TO ACTIVATE
ABDOMINAL MUSCLES

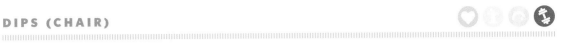

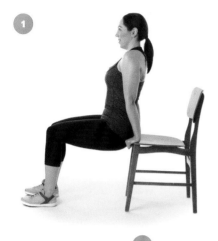

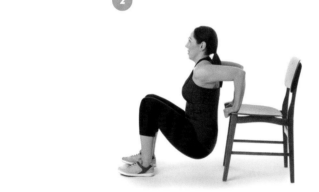

1 Find a stable chair or park bench. Hold on to the edge of the seat with your hands shoulder-width apart. Stretch your legs out in front (straight or bent).

2 Lower your body so there is a 90-degree angle between the upper arm and forearm.

3 With arms at a right angle, press down through your palms, lifting the upper body back into starting position. Keep your elbows tight, paying close attention not to allow them to flare out as this will place stress on the shoulders and elbows.

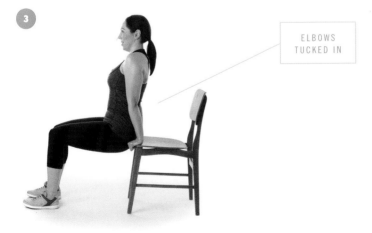

ELBOWS TUCKED IN

1 Step one foot forward.

2 Bring the second foot to meet
the first foot, then return the
first foot to its starting position and the second foot to
meet the first foot. Repeat.

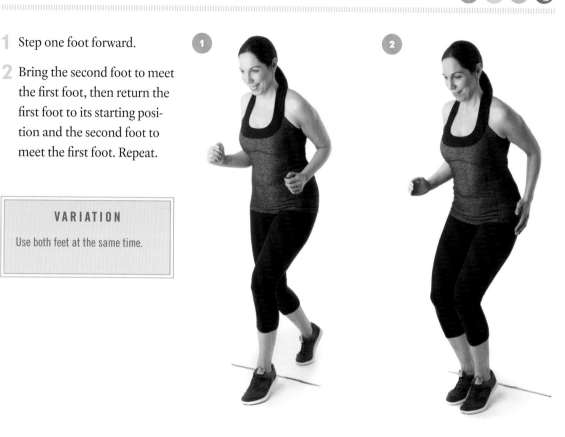

VARIATION

Use both feet at the same time.

> **It does not matter how
> slowly you go as long as
> you do not stop.**
> —CONFUCIUS

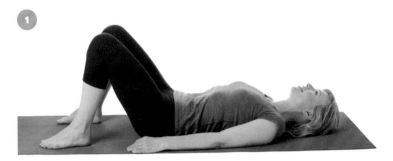

1 Lie on your back with your knees bent and feet flat, hip-width apart and close to your bottom. Keep your arms close to your body, your hands outstretched, palms facing down.

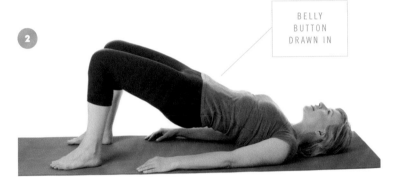

BELLY BUTTON DRAWN IN

2 Push into your feet as you raise your hips off the ground, one vertebra at a time while activating your glutes.

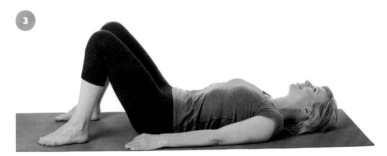

3 Hold for a few seconds, then return your hips to the ground in preparation for the next rep.

KEY POINTS

» Don't hyperextend your back.
» Keep your knees pointing toward the ceiling—don't let them cave inwards.
» Squeeze those glutes.

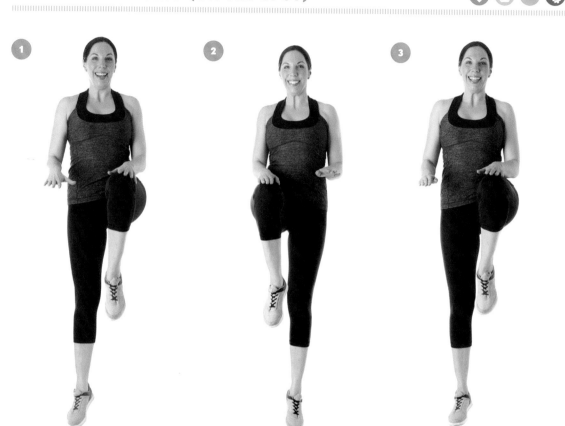

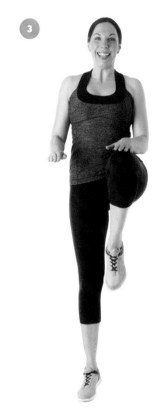

1 Do a light jog on the spot.

2 Place your hands out, your elbows bent at 90 degrees.

3 While jogging, lift your knees higher, so that your thighs reach 90 degrees and aim to touch your hands.

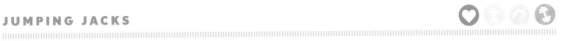

1

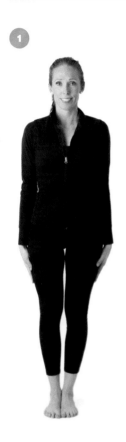

3

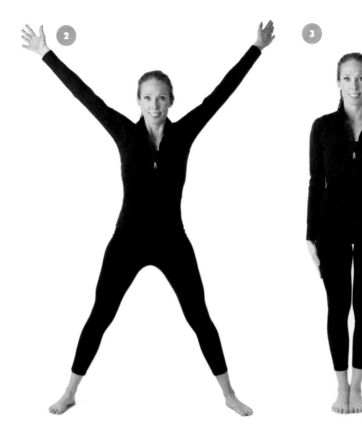

1 Start as if you're standing at attention—arms down by your side, legs together.

2 Jump your feet and spread your arms out wide.

3 Jump back to the starting position and repeat.

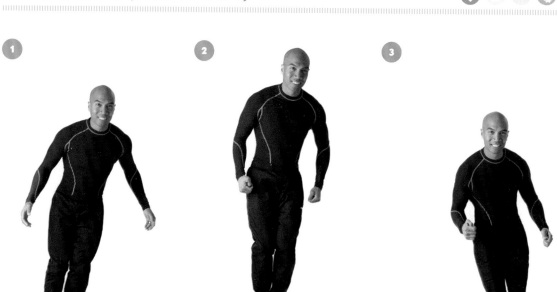

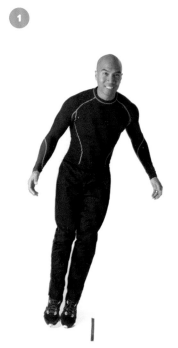

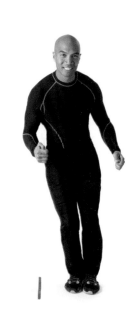

1 Imagine a line on the floor; stand on one side of it. Bring your feet together, arms bent at your side. Bend slightly forward at the hips and the knees.

2 Keeping your core tight, jump to the other side of the line.

3 Keep your feet together while hopping sideways back and forth over the line—like a slalom skier.

VARIATION

Jump with a single foot.

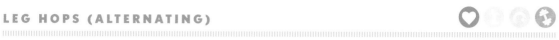

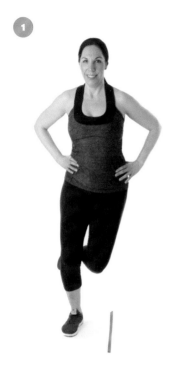

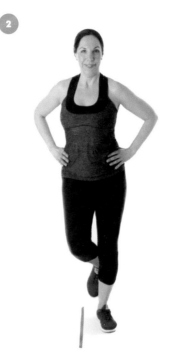

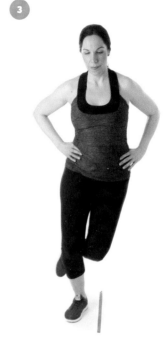

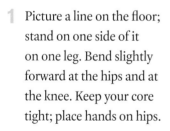

1 Picture a line on the floor; stand on one side of it on one leg. Bend slightly forward at the hips and at the knee. Keep your core tight; place hands on hips.

2 Hop across the line onto the ball of your other foot.

3 Switch legs back and forth repeatedly, based on allotted time/sets/reps.

KEY POINT

» These are small jumps, done reasonably quickly.

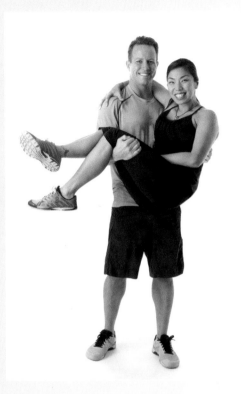

"After I suffered an injury in hockey, I stopped playing and I went up to 32 per cent body fat. So, three years ago, I turned to the most fit guy I know for help: Dai Manuel. Slowly I worked at getting into the shape I'm in today." —OWEN

"As a social worker and busy mother of four, I have to keep mentally and physically fit, so I like to mix up my movements. I practise ashtanga yoga as well as CrossFit and Whole Life Fitness Power 30 whenever I can." —EVELYN

"I danced as a child, but when I went to college I lost interest in fitness because I felt intimidated by gyms and was afraid to go to a class by myself. I was invited to join the Sunday Funday Throwdowns with Dai and Christie and have felt so comfortable working out with such a supportive community. Physically and mentally I am a new person since committing to the Whole Life Fitness Power 30." —GEORGINA

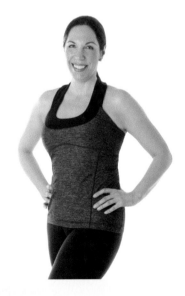

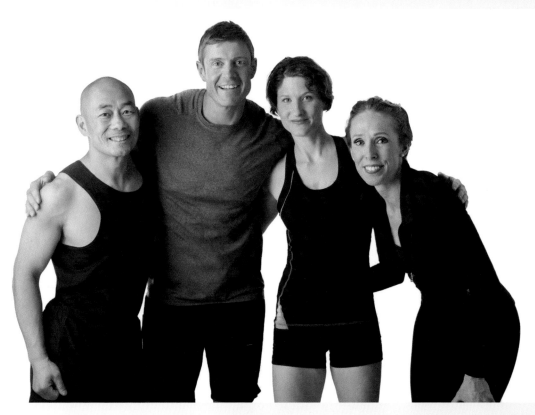

"In 2006, I was hit by a truck while I was riding my bicycle, which left me with numerous broken bones, including my pelvis. I was in a body cast for six months without the ability to exercise. Slowly, I returned to running and, while I am not fast, I find that movement is the best medicine. Without exercise, my life would be very painful."
—ALLISON

"I've always played team sports, such as volleyball and rugby, and I love hiking with my family. I just know that to really enjoy life to the fullest, I need to be fit." —JOHN

"I was involved in athletic activities all my life. I have always struggled with traditional gyms though, so when I was introduced to FUN-ctional fitness through high-intensity CrossFit training, I was thrilled with the results and motivated to continue. An entrepreneur and busy mom, I need something that's efficient and keeps me stimulated and healthy for years to come. The Whole Life Fitness Power 30 has helped me be healthier, inside and out, and the community keeps me coming back!" —CHRISTIE

1 Start in neutral stance with hands on your hips.

2 Step one foot forward about half a body's length. Make sure the front shin is as upright as possible and the knee does not go past the toes. The back knee lowers to the ground, allowing the knee to lightly touch the floor—just as you would give a kiss on a baby's cheek— it's not a smacker!

3 Press the weight through the front heel. Keep upper body upright. Press into the front heel to fire back to starting position. Switch legs and repeat.

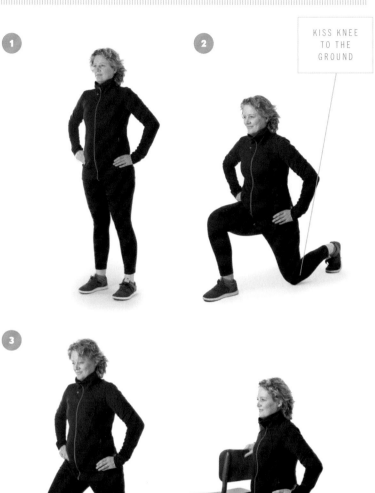

KISS KNEE TO THE GROUND

KEY POINT:

» You are not on a tightrope, so ensure your feet remain hip-width apart when you step forward.

VARIATION:

Use a chair for stability.

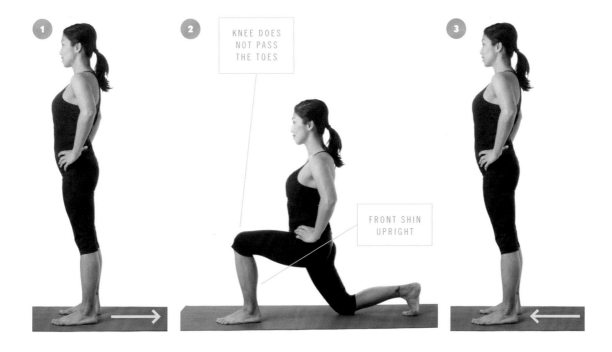

KNEE DOES NOT PASS THE TOES

FRONT SHIN UPRIGHT

1 Start in neutral stance with hands on your hips or at your side.

2 Step one foot back about half a body's length, making sure the front shin is as upright as possible and the knee does not go past the toes. Lower the back knee to the ground, allowing the knee to lightly touch the floor.

3 Press your weight through the front heel, keeping your core engaged and upper body upright. Press through the back foot to fire back up and forward returning to the starting position (neutral stance). Repeat with other leg.

KEY POINT

» Reverse lunges are recommended if you have bad knees.

1 Start in neutral stance. Bend your knees slightly and tilt forward at your hips.

2 Step your left food behind your right leg and bend both knees to lower your body into a lunge. Move your left knee behind your right heel, allowing your right arm to mirror your right leg. Keeping your front foot firmly planted, lower your back knee to gently touch the floor.

3 Return to starting position.

4 Switch legs and repeat.

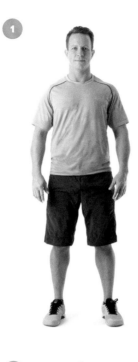

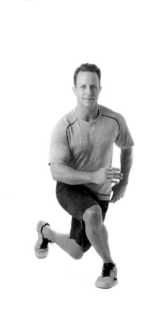

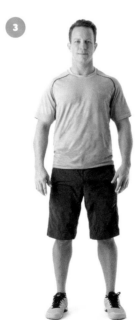

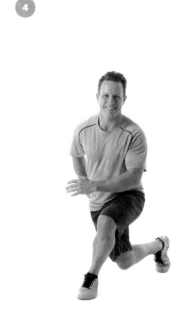

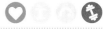

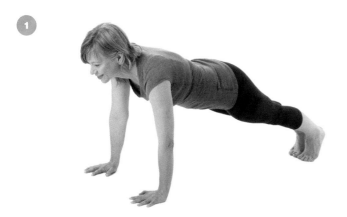

1 Start in plank position with arms fully extended. Engage your core.

2 Bring your right foot forward, as close to the outside of your right hand as possible.

3 Quickly pop the hip up slightly, as you fire your right leg back to the starting position. Switch your legs, bringing the left forward to the outside of your left hand and returning your left leg to the starting position.

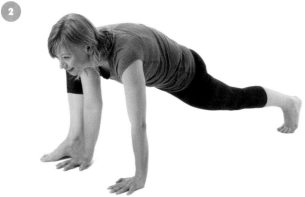

KEY POINTS

» Keep your core rock solid.
» Alternate left and right legs.
» Speed of the legs will vary depending on ability.

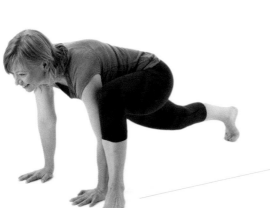

FOOT IN LINE WITH HAND

STRAIGHT ARM PLANK

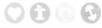

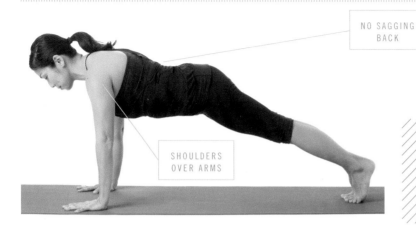

NO SAGGING BACK

SHOULDERS OVER ARMS

KEY POINT

» When planking keep a neutral neck

1 Lie flat on your tummy. Place hands under your shoulders, elbows into your sides. Pull your core in.

2 Extend your arms, lifting your body and legs off the ground; make sure there is no sagging or overarching in the back. Palms of your hands and balls of your feet are your only contacts to the ground.

STANDARD FRONT PLANK (FROM ELBOWS)

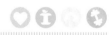

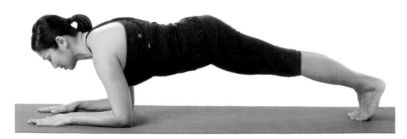

1 Lie flat on your tummy. Lift your body up onto your forearms, which should be shoulder-width apart.

2 Engage your core. Keep your shoulders directly over your elbows; make sure there is no sagging or over-arching in the back. Knees and forearms are your only contacts with the ground.

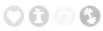

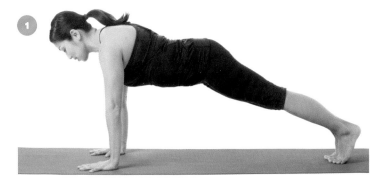

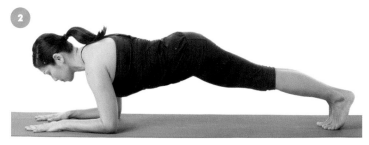

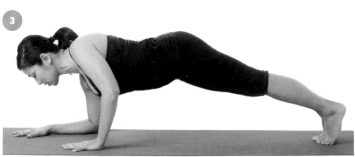

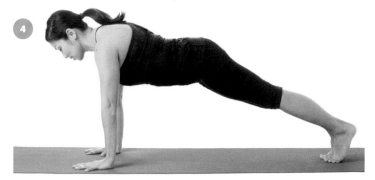

1 Start in straight arm plank position.

2 Engage your core. Lower yourself to the ground into the standard front plank position from the elbows.

3 Raise the left side of your body by pressing your left hand firmly down and into the floor and straighten your arm.

4 Do the same with your right side, returning to a straight arm plank position. Repeat by alternating between arms i.e., down left, down right, up left, up right, then down right, down left, up right, up left, etc.

VARIATION

For greater intensity, stack one foot on top of the other, or alternate raising one leg at a time.

1 Lie on your right side in a straight line from head to feet. Rest on your forearm. Elbow should be directly underneath your shoulder. Contract your core muscles, and lift your right hip up off the floor while maintaining a nice straight line with your body from ankles to shoulders. Rest your other arm and your foot on your body, stacking your feet together. Hold this position for the set time. Switch sides.

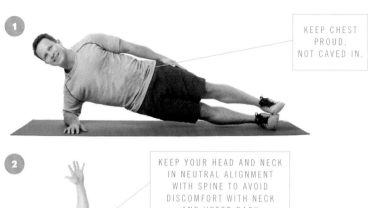

KEEP CHEST PROUD, NOT CAVED IN.

2 Lift arm straight up in the air, maintaining a nice straight line.

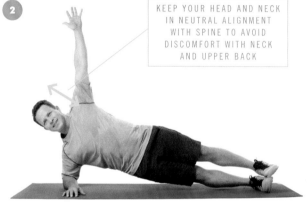

KEEP YOUR HEAD AND NECK IN NEUTRAL ALIGNMENT WITH SPINE TO AVOID DISCOMFORT WITH NECK AND UPPER BACK

3 To modify this movement, use your foot to assist with lifting and supporting your body's weight while in plank position. Place the top foot flat on the floor (positioning somewhere between the knee and supporting foot.) Press down through the supporting foot while in side plank position.

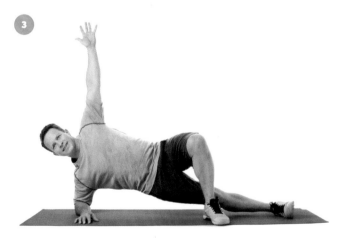

VARIATION

Rest on your knees instead of your feet.

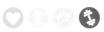

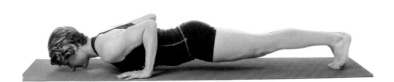

1. Lie flat on the floor with your face to the ground. Engage your core and glutes. Hands beneath your shoulders, legs together. Your palms, chest and toes are the only points of contact with the ground.

SHOULDERS TO ANKLES = STRAIGHT LINE

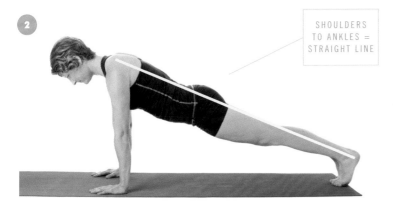

2. Press up until arms are straight. Keep in a straight line from shoulder to ankle.

3. Lower body until chest touches the mat. Push back up to straighten arms again.

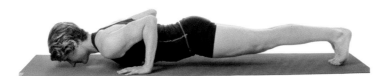

KEY POINTS

» Keep elbows as close to your body as possible.
» Ideally you go from three points (hands, chest, toes) of contact to two points (hands, toes), back to three and then two, and so on.

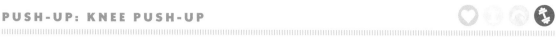

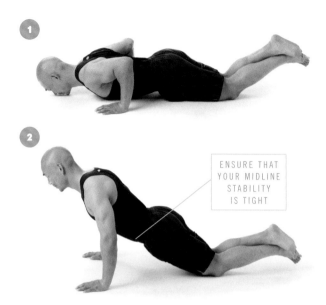

1 Lie on the floor with hands positioned under shoulders. Knees, chest and palms should be only parts of body in contact with floor. (Make sure to have thighs, hips, stomach off floor.)

2 Bend knees and raise body up off floor by extending your arms while maintaining a straight body. Lower body until chest touches the floor.

ENSURE THAT YOUR MIDLINE STABILITY IS TIGHT

PUSH-UP: WALL PUSH-UP

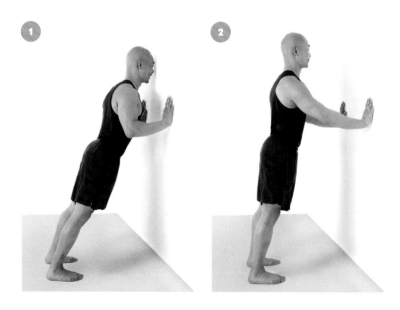

1 Face a wall (or a stable chair or countertop) in neutral stance. Lean body forward, placing hands on the wall at roughly shoulder height. Lower upper body towards the wall, gently touch nose against wall surface.

2 Press through palms, pushing your upper body up and away from the wall until arms are straight. Repeat for desired repetitive range.

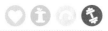

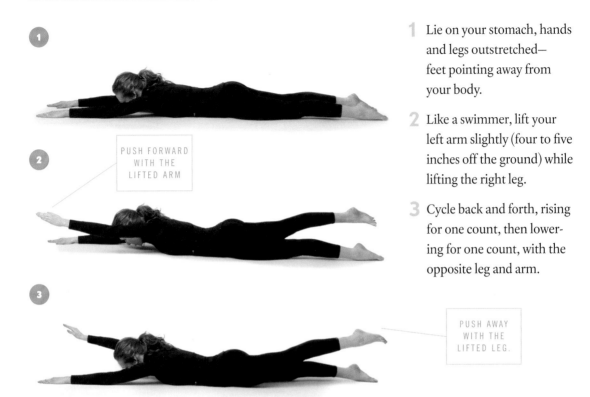

PUSH FORWARD WITH THE LIFTED ARM

PUSH AWAY WITH THE LIFTED LEG.

1 Lie on your stomach, hands and legs outstretched—feet pointing away from your body.

2 Like a swimmer, lift your left arm slightly (four to five inches off the ground) while lifting the right leg.

3 Cycle back and forth, rising for one count, then lowering for one count, with the opposite leg and arm.

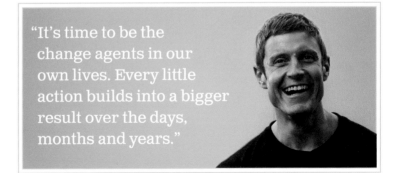

"It's time to be the change agents in our own lives. Every little action builds into a bigger result over the days, months and years."

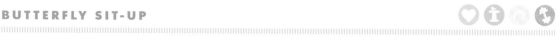

1 Sit on the floor with your knees bent out to the sides and the soles of your feet pressed against each other. Press your knees down to the floor. Extend your body back to the floor, hands above your head.

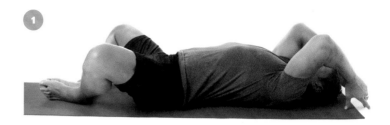

2 Use your upper body to propel yourself forward until you are sitting up, your arms between your legs as you touch your toes.

3 Return to the floor and repeat.

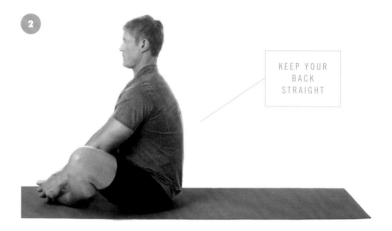

KEEP YOUR
BACK
STRAIGHT

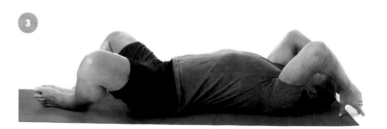

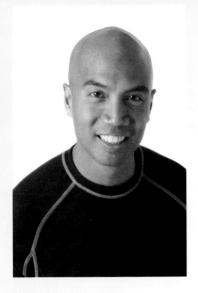

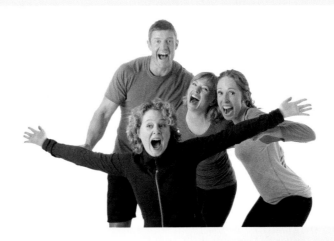

"My motivation stems from a belief that was instilled in me by my brother and father, that we should all get stronger with age. I am determined to live a healthy lifestyle so I can enjoy my passion for art and photography and take care of my beautiful wife and children. It is important for me to surround myself with wonderful people like Dai, Christie and the whole Sunday Funday family as they share the same healthy beliefs and lifestyle." —RON

"I've always dabbled with fitness—from Jane Fonda-style aerobics in the 80s and 90s to yoga and Zumba and TRX. I'm just keen on keeping flexible as I age and with an erratic life as a freelancer, I'm always keen to save time and keep fit wherever I am. The Whole Life Fitness Power 30 has spurred me into daily action—no matter where I am traveling for my job." —LUCY

"In the past, I thought working out had to mean high-intensity, high-impact aerobic exercise. My body doesn't like that kind of activity—I get dizzy and exhausted quickly, so I would tend to avoid it altogether, and then feel really guilty about it. Now I just do the kind of exercise I enjoy—a lot of yoga, and Dai's Whole Life Fitness Power 30. This kind of workout suits my body and my lifestyle, so it's easy to keep it up for the long haul." —MAGGIE

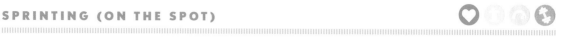

1 Jog lightly on the spot.

2 Bend your torso slightly forward, keeping your weight on your toes and sprint fast while pumping your arms close to your body as fast as you can.

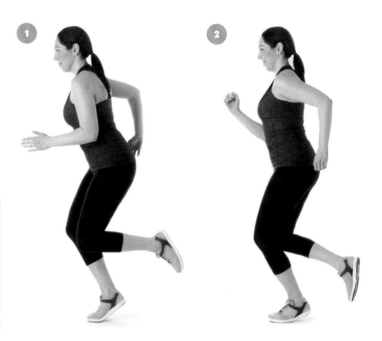

KEY POINTS

» Stay on your toes.
» Pick a spot about a body's length in front of you to focus on.

"It's not what we do once in a while that shapes our lives. It's what we do consistently."

—ANTHONY ROBBINS

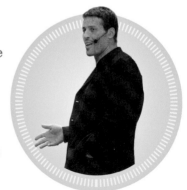

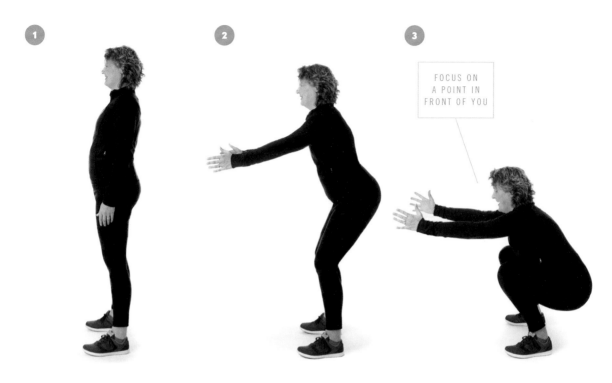

FOCUS ON
A POINT IN
FRONT OF YOU

1 Start in neutral stance and push your bottom backwards, weight into your heels.

2 With your arms outstretched in front of you, bend your knees.

3 Sink your hips below your knee height, keeping your knees above or behind your toes.

KEY POINTS

» Widen your stance if you have limited hip mobility.
» Point toes out slightly and push your knees out if they begin to cave inwards.

VARIATION

Use a countertop or railing for balance.

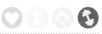

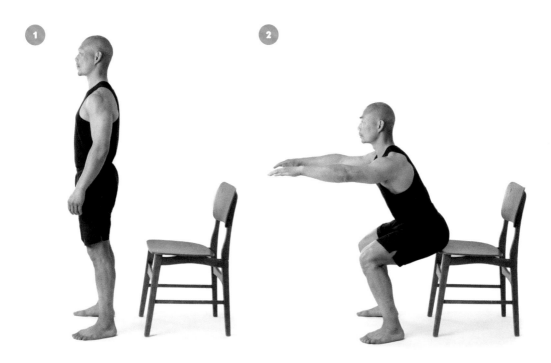

1 Place a chair behind you and perform a standard squat (page 121).

2 Allow your bottom to lightly touch the seat of the chair.

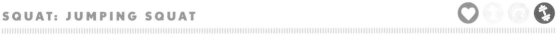

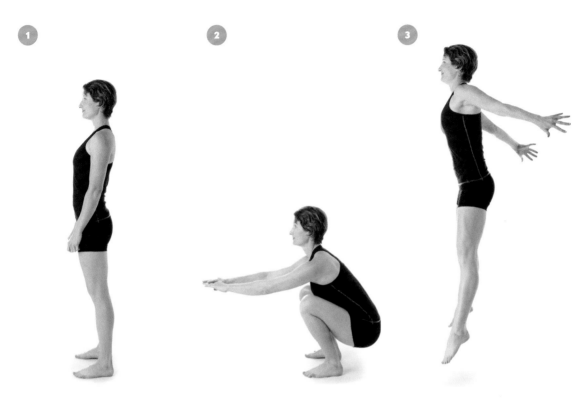

1 Start in neutral stance.

2 Perform a standard squat (page 121) Push your weight down into the floor.

3 Thrust upward, extending your body into the air and opening your hips at the top.

KEY POINT

» Keep your knees bent as you enter the landing position (page 90).

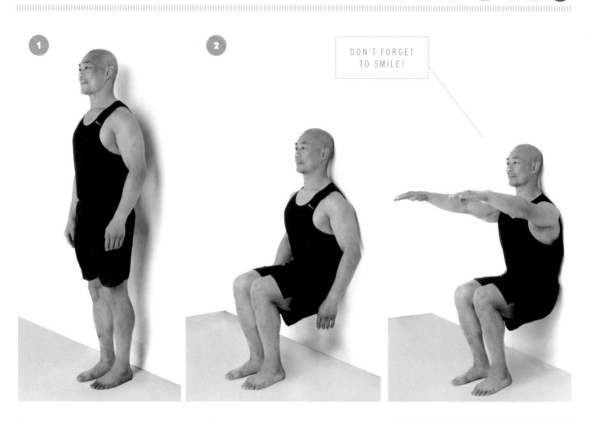

DON'T FORGET
TO SMILE!

1 Stand against a wall with back flat against it.

2 With feet about hip-width apart, place your feet about 45 cm (18 in) from the wall. Lower your body until your legs are at a right angle (90 degrees).

3 Hold this position for the set time.

VARIATION

To add a little spice to this move, raise your arms up to shoulder height, in front of you.

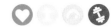

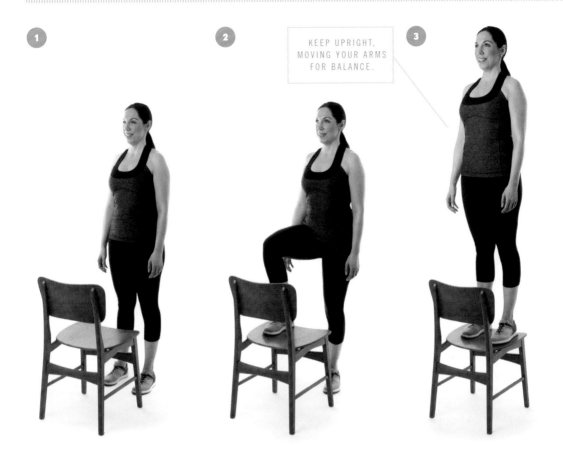

KEEP UPRIGHT,
MOVING YOUR ARMS
FOR BALANCE.

1 Start in neutral stance, facing a chair, stair or bench.

2 Place your right foot on the chair, with your right knee at a right angle.

3 Straighten your right leg as you raise your left foot to the chair. Keep upright, moving your arms for balance. Step down with your right foot, then your left to starting position.

KEY POINTS

» Land on the ball of your foot.
» Be sure to alternate the leading leg.

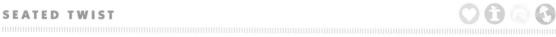

1 Start seated on the floor, back straight, legs together and knees slightly bent. Keeping legs together, raise your feet slightly off the ground; core engaged.

2 Bend your arms and twist your torso to one side, keeping your legs still.

3 Now twist your arms and torso to the other side. Continue, alternating left and right side twists.

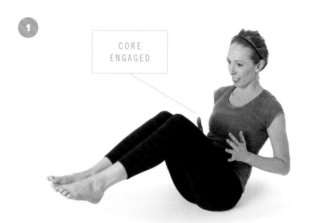

CORE ENGAGED

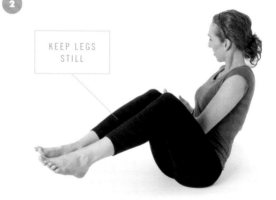

KEEP LEGS STILL

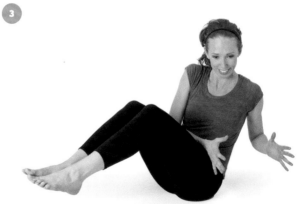

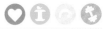

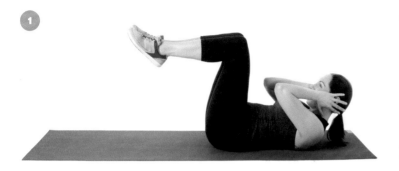

1 Lie on your back and elevate knees to 90 degrees. Bring your hands lightly to your temple, elbows bent. Raise your head slightly off the ground.

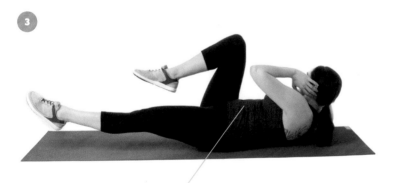

2 Bending your left knee toward your chest, rotate your right elbow towards your left knee, while extending your right leg closer to the floor.

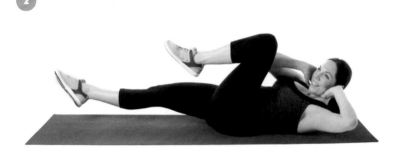

3 Extend your left leg while releasing your right arm and bending your right knee toward your chest to meet your left elbow. Continue alternating right and left connection.

KEY POINTS

» Imagine that you are riding a bike.
» Core remains engaged the entire time.

ENGAGED CORE

1 LIVE A LIFE
FULL OF
VICTORIES

#WLFMANIFESTO

2 LIVE
THROUGH
ACTION

*The day you stop moving
is the day you stop living*

3 INVEST DAILY
INTO YOUR

**HEALTH &
FITNESS**

*YOUR ROI IS A LIFETIME
OF AWESOMENESS!*

12 BE A ROLE MODEL AND LEAD BY EXAMPLE

REPLACE WORDS LIKE

I THINK
WITH
I CAN

WILL TRY
WITH
I DO

AND, MOST IMPORTANTLY, JUST DO IT WITH **#JUSTDIDIT**

4 DO SHORT
INTENSE
WORKOUTS

THAT PROVIDE
RESULTS

11 FIND AN
ACCOMPLISHMENT
TO **CELEBRATE**

NO GUILT.
SHAME.
BLAME.

13 WHOLE LIFE
FITNESS MANIFESTO

"**WORKOUT
ON YOUR
OWN,
BUT NEVER
ALONE.**"

5 **DON'T
OBSESS**

ABOUT THE SCALE (IT IS JUST A NUMBER)

GO BY FEEL!
REMEMBER **STRONG
& HEALTHY** EQUALS
THE **NEW SKINNY**

10 **WE ARE
COMMUNITY:**
HONOUR THY
TRIBE.

WE CELEBRATE OUR **WINS**,
CONSOLE OUR LOSSES, **HOLD**
EACH OTHER **ACCOUNTABLE** AND
SHARE IN A COMMON
DESIRE TO BE **AWESOME**.

6 LACK OF TIME, TOO TIRED
& NOT KNOWING HOW TO
DO IT ARE JUST EXCUSES.

REPLACE EXCUSES WITH
THE MANTRA:
**THERE'S NO SUCH THING AS
EXCUSES, JUST BAD HABITS
IN DISGUISE**

9 **NO** EQUIPMENT
PROBLEM!

MY BODY
IS THE ONLY PIECE
OF EQUIPMENT I NEED

I HONOUR & RESPECT
MY BODY FOR LIFE

8 **THE 2%
SOLUTION**

"DO WHAT YOU CAN,
WHEN YOU CAN, AND DON'T
LET LACK OF TIME BE YOUR
EXCUSE - EVERYONE HAS
30 MINUTES A DAY"

7 **LIVE
A LIFE**

OF AWESOMENESS AND HELP
OTHERS IN DOING THE SAME...
ALWAYS AND ANY WAY

WE CAN

THE WHOLE LIFE FITNESS POWER 30

CHAPTER 8

FOR ANY POSITIVE CHANGE TO be sustainable, it has to become a habit. That's why it helps to have a program to follow, especially at first. Once your healthy habits are well ingrained, you can go freestyle with your fitness. By that point, you will have internalized the great feeling you get from moving your body regularly, and it will be much easier to know what you need to do in order to feel the way you want to feel. Until that magic moment, we've got you covered with a powerful four-week plan: 30 minutes of movement, mindfulness and personal development a day, every day, for four weeks.

THE POWER OF 30 MINUTES A DAY

1. 15 minutes for your workout of the day (WOD)
2. Five minutes for mindful meditation
3. 10 minutes for personal development

I've structured this program this way simply because in working with clients over the years, I have seen that many people find four weeks to be a great time frame for forming a new, lasting habit. But you won't want to stop there! This program is totally flexible and meant to last a lifetime. Once your initial four weeks are up, you may wish to commit to doing the four weeks again, making adjustments or adding new elements that suit you.

Your results will really depend on how much you embrace your new routine, and whether you do so with integrity. By continually repeating good patterns of behaviour over days, weeks and months, you will inevitably begin to feel the benefits. And, as you know by now, feeling great is the best motivator to keep going strong.

> " Dai Manuel is one of the most genuine, positive and inspiring people I know. Dai encourages others to lead a healthy lifestyle and does so inclusively, regardless of a person's physical ability or fitness level. It's truly a joy to witness the growth in others due to the support of Dai and his family." —CHERYL

WARM UP

It's important to prepare your body before a workout. Your warm-up routine should take five to 10 minutes, before your workout of the day. You won't need much space—in fact, warm-ups work just great in a living room, small gym or even a hotel room. Feel your core temperature rise and your heart rate increase as you start to sweat a little. Cycle through these exercises one or two times. Enjoy!

Jog on the spot: 30 to 60 seconds

Feet shuffle, over and back: 30 seconds

Lateral hops side-to-side: 30 seconds

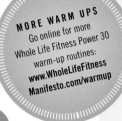

MORE WARM UPS Go online for more Whole Life Fitness Power 30 warm-up routines: www.WholeLifeFitness Manifesto.com/warmup

Jumping jacks: 30 to 60 seconds

Lunge with a twist: 8 to 10 reps per side

Side plank: 30 seconds per side

COOL DOWN

Why cool down after a workout? In a nutshell, it just feels good to relax the heart, unwind and calm down your breathing. It's a good way to flush some of the lactic acid out of your muscles and to help bring down the heart rate as well. This cool-down/recovery routine takes from 15 to 30 minutes. Don't worry if you don't have time to do it all every time. Just follow these suggestions when you can.

 Try 5 to 10 minutes of easy walking/rowing/cycling

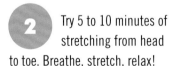 Try 5 to 10 minutes of stretching from head to toe. Breathe, stretch, relax!

Try 5 to 10 minutes of SMR (self myofascial release), breaking up of knots in the muscles/fascia, with either a roller or a lacrosse/tennis ball.

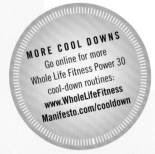

MORE COOL DOWNS Go online for more Whole Life Fitness Power 30 cool-down routines: www.WholeLifeFitness Manifesto.com/cooldown

To get the most out of the Whole Life Fitness Power 30:

- Take pictures of your food and beverages.
- Join our online community at www.WholeLifeFitnessManifesto.com. Be sure to post photos, feedback and testimonials.
- Cultivate an "all-in" mentality. You are part of a team! We are here to support each other toward reaching our goals.

To Do List and Next Steps:

1. Review the basic moves for the four-week Whole Life Fitness Power 30 program in Chapter 7.
2. Fill out your goals and measurements using the charts on page 133, or online at www.WholeLifeFitnessManifesto.com/Goals andMeasurements.
3. Complete the baseline fitness test on page 135. (Please feel free to submit your score—in confidence—to coach@wholelifefitnessmanifesto.com.)
4. Take your before photos (bathing suit or shorts/sport bra recommended—the more skin the better), including head-to-toe of your front, back, profile left, profile right in a well-lit space. (You can share these or keep them private, but believe me you will be glad you have them down the road.)
5. Get ready to crush it!

FORMING HABITS

How long does it take to establish a new habit? Once you get started, how long should it take for a new routine to start to feel normal—a week, a month, a year? There are many different points of view on this. Some say it takes 21 days, others indicate it might take longer. But why is there so much conflicting info about the actual length of time it takes to form a habit? Back in 1960, Dr. Maxwell Maltz published a book called Psycho-Cybernetics, in which he stated that amputees took on average 21 days to adjust to losing a limb. He noted that most people need at least 21 days to adjust to any major life changes (another way of thinking of habits).

Dr. Maltz's findings were very influential within the self-help community, including personal development coaches Brian Tracy, Zig Ziglar and Anthony Robbins. The statistic has been thrown around a little too literally by some people since then. But Maltz noted that it takes a minimum of 21 days, not "it takes 21 days." In 2009 Phillippa Lally performed a study focusing on "How Habits are Formed." Her study went on to find that those that participated took anywhere from 18 to 254 days to get to the point where they were automatic with performing the actions (habits), but the average was 66 days.

RECORD YOUR SMART FITNESS GOALS

STEP 1

PICK A SPECIFIC GOAL
Why this goal? Make it SMART—specific, measurable, actionable, realistic, and time-sensitive.

STEP 2

MEASURE YOUR GOAL
List a couple of ways you can measure your goal, for example, how quickly you want to complete a 5-km race, a specific outfit you want to wear, etc.

STEP 3

MAKE YOUR GOAL ACTIONABLE
What actions are you going to take to ensure that you complete your goal? For instance, will you give up sugar or alcohol, and commit to completing all four weeks of the Whole Life Fitness Power 30?

STEP 4

BE REALISTIC
Can your goal be reached in your chosen timeframe?

STEP 5

WHAT'S YOUR TIMEFRAME?
What is the specific date of your race, hot date, or other special experience? How will you celebrate achieving your goal?

To fill these worksheets out online, go to www.WholeLifeFitnessManifesto.com/goalsandmeasurements.

MEASUREMENTS

Write down your physical measurements before and after the four-week program

BEFORE

Neck: _____ inches
(measured mid-neck)

Upper arm: _____ inches
(measured at armpit)

Chest/bust: _____ inches
(measured at nipple)

Waist: _____ inches
(measured at belly button)

Hips: _____ inches
(measured at hip bone)

Thigh: _____ inches
(measured at mid-thigh)

Calf: _____ inches
(measured at mid-calf)

Weight: _____ pounds

AFTER

Neck: _____ inches
(measured mid-neck)

Upper arm: _____ inches
(measured at armpit)

Chest/bust: _____ inches
(measured at nipple)

Waist: _____ inches
(measured at belly button)

Hips: _____ inches
(measured at hip bone)

Thigh: _____ inches
(measured at mid-thigh)

Calf: _____ inches
(measured at mid-calf)

Weight: _____ pounds

To fill these worksheets out online, go to www.WholeLifeFitnessManifesto.com/goalsandmeasurements

BASELINE FITNESS TESTING

In order to track your progress, you need to have a clear picture of where you're starting out. This baseline fitness test is based on the 10 components of physical fitness, as defined by Jim Crawley and Bruce Evans.

1. **Cardiovascular/Respiratory Endurance:** The body's ability to collect, process and deliver oxygen.
2. **Stamina:** The body's ability to process, deliver, store and use energy.
3. **Strength:** The ability of a muscle or groups of muscles to apply force.
4. **Flexibility:** The ability to maximize the range of motion of a given joint.
5. **Power:** The ability of a group of muscles to apply great force in a short window of time.
6. **Speed:** The ability to reduce the time frame of a repeated movement.
7. **Coordination:** The ability to combine several distinct movement patterns into a single distinct movement.
8. **Agility:** The ability to decrease transition time from one movement pattern to another.
9. **Balance:** The ability to control the placement of the body's centre of gravity in relation to its support base.
10. **Accuracy:** The ability to control movement in a given direction or at a given intensity.

SELF-GUIDED TESTING PROTOCOL

GOAL OF TESTING: To establish a score that provides insight into our present state of health as it relates to the 10 components of fitness.

1

TAKE TEST

2

RECORD SCORES FOR
FUTURE REFERENCE

3

REPEAT BASELINE ONCE
EVERY 8 WEEKS

BASIC BASELINE FITNESS TEST

SQUATS	How many can you complete in 1 minute?	Basic movement or a modified variation?
PUSH-UPS	How many can you complete in 1 minute?	Basic movement or a modified variation?
SIT-UPS	How many can you complete in 1 minute?	Basic movement or a modified variation?
1 MILE* JOG / RUN	How many minutes did it take to complete?	
STORK BALANCE	How many seconds can you stand on one leg?	
SIT & REACH	Sit with your legs extended in front of you. Bend from your waist. How far can you reach toward (or beyond) your toes?	

* Find a 1.6 km (1-mile) track, use a treadmill, or use the "Map My Run" app to chart a 1-mile course.
Be sure to use the same course or method when re-testing at the end of the four-week program!

Want to dig deeper into your own stats? You'll find a more comprehensive version of the baseline fitness test at www.WholeLifeFitnessManifesto.com/baseline

> " Even though I didn't really do much running, I reduced my time from 13:31 to 11:51, scoring a 12.5% improvement!"
>
> —JASON

Week 1 is about creating some new habits, and taking stock of our challenges. Throughout the week, strive to incorporate the following habits:

1. Drink two to three litres of water each day.
2. Avoid soft drinks, fruit juices and alcohol on weekdays.
3. Eat more greens, fruits and whole foods. Eat less processed or pre-packaged foods.
4. Recognize a simple accomplishment at the end of each day and share it via social networking (#WLFManifesto), or in a journal.
5. Walk with your head held proud and make eye contact, offering a smile to those you meet. Believe YOU are AWESOME, period.

EVERY DAY

✔ Drink two glasses of **water** upon waking.

✔ Complete a **warm-up** (optional, but recommended).

✔ **15-minute WOD** (workout of the day), as many rounds or repetitions as possible (AMRAP).

✔ Finish with a **cool-down** (optional, but recommended).

✔ Five minutes **meditation**: stillness, reflection and thankfulness.

✔ 10 minutes **personal development**. Feed your mind. Read, write, listen to inspiring ideas and information.

15-MIN WOD EXERCISES

DAY-BY-DAY BREAKDOWN

When you finish one set of each exercise, start over until you reach the 15-minute mark. (And don't forget to record your score—how many rounds did you do?)

DAY 1
1. 5 × push-ups
2. 10 × sit-ups
3. 15 × squats

DAY 2
1. 10 × alternating reverse lunges (5 per leg)
2. 40 × air-skips

DAY 3
1. 15 × chair squats
2. 15 × chair step-ups
3. 15 × chair dips
4. 15 × wall push-ups

DAY 4
1. 20-second sprint (on the spot)
2. 20-second rest
3. 20 seconds jumping jacks
4. 20-second rest

DAY 5
1. 30 seconds chair/bench step-ups
2. 30 seconds push-ups
3. 30-second plank
4. 30-second rest

DAY 6
1. 15 × glute bridges
2. 45-second plank
3. 15-30 seconds rest

DAY 7
1. 7 × burpees
2. 30-second rest

DAILY CHECKLIST

Use this checklist to help you organize your week.

Download a printable version from wholelifefitnessmanifesto.com/resources.

TO DO:	DRINK 2 TO 3L OF WATER	15 MINUTE WOD	5 MINUTES OF MINDFULNESS	10 MINUTES OF PERSONAL DEVELOPMENT	NO POP, NO ALCOHOL, NO PROBLEM	EAT MORE FRUIT & VEGGIES	SHARE MY AWESOMENESS WITH FRIENDS
Sunday							
Monday							
Tuesday							
Wednesday							
Thursday							
Friday							
Saturday							

AND SO COMPLETES WEEK 1. BOO—YAH!

JOURNAL

Use this page for your victories, challenges, suggestions,
comments and emotions.

Download a printable version from wholelifefitnessmanifesto.com/resources.

HOW DID IT GO?

» What am I proud
of accomplishing?

» What did I find easy
or hard?

» What personal
development am
I enjoying?

WEEK 2

In Week 2, you're going to continue to build on your momentum from Week 1. By now you are feeling the benefits of making time for you, and realizing you are capable of making real change in your life. Hopefully, you are noticing some changes in mood, energy, stress levels and muscle tone, as well as new surges of creativity, productivity and awesomeness—a direct byproduct of your 30-minute Whole Life Fitness Power 30 ritual.

A few things to shoot for this week:

1. Drink two to three litres of water each day.
2. Limit yourself to five "treat" beverages (soft drinks, juice, and alcohol) throughout the entire week.
3. Aim to incorporate GREEN with every meal (bonus points for incorporating more than just a green garnish).
4. Compliment a different person each day.

EVERY DAY

- ✔ Drink two glasses of **water** upon waking.
- ✔ Complete a **warm-up** (optional, but recommended).
- ✔ **15-minute WOD** (workout of the day), as many rounds or repetitions as possible (AMRAP).
- ✔ Finish with a **cool-down** (optional, but recommended).
- ✔ Five minutes **meditation**: stillness, reflection and thankfulness.
- ✔ 10 minutes **personal development**. Feed your mind. Read, write, listen to inspiring ideas and information.

15-MIN WOD EXERCISES

DAY-BY-DAY BREAKDOWN

When you finish one set of each exercise, start over until you reach the 15-minute mark. (And don't forget to record your score—how many rounds did you do?)

DAY 8

1. 50 × air skips
2. 25 × crunches/sit-ups

DAY 9

1. 10 × caterpillar stretches
2. 30-second squat hold (keep legs at a right angle; a wall sit is perfect!)

DAY 10

1. 50 × jumping jacks
2. 40 × squats
3. 30 × sit-ups/crunches
4. 20 × push-ups
5. 10 × burpees

DAY 11

1. Walk 60–90 seconds outdoors. (Indoors: brisk march on the spot for 60–90 seconds)
2. Jog 15–30 seconds. (Indoors: knee-raises to hip height, moderate pacing for 15–30 seconds)
3. Run 5–15 seconds. (Indoors: fast feet, sprint on spot with high knees for 5–15 seconds)

DAY 12

1. 30 seconds lateral hops (side-to-side)
2. 30 seconds feet shuffle
3. 30 seconds jumping jacks
4. 30-second rest

DAY 13

1. 30-second front plank
2. 30-second right side plank
3. 30-second left side plank
4. 60-second rest

DAY 14

1. 10 × burpees
2. 30-second plank

DAILY CHECKLIST

Use this checklist to help you organize your week.

Download a printable version from wholelifefitnessmanifesto.com/resources.

TO DO:	DRINK 2 TO 3L OF WATER	15 MINUTE WOD	5 MINUTES OF MINDFULNESS	10 MINUTES OF PERSONAL DEVELOPMENT	NO POP, NO ALCOHOL, NO PROBLEM	EAT MORE FRUIT & VEGGIES	COMPLIMENT SOMEONE
Sunday							
Monday							
Tuesday							
Wednesday							
Thursday							
Friday							
Saturday							

AND SO COMPLETES WEEK 2. **BAM!**

JOURNAL

Use this page for your victories, challenges, suggestions, comments and emotions.

Download a printable version from wholelifefitnessmanifesto.com/resources.

HOW DID IT GO?

» How have my energy levels changed?
» Who did I reach out to with kind words?
» What am I enjoying about mindfulness?

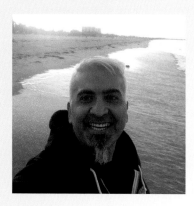
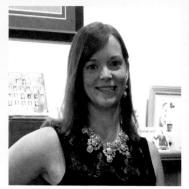
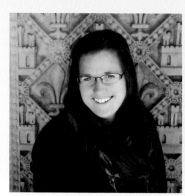

“Positive influence, friend, caring, generous, on a mission, life enhancer, supportive—take your pick—Dai Manuel is all of that. He first got my attention on social media. I thought: This guy practises what he preaches, and that's rare these days. My life has truly been set on a better path because of Dai's guidance. He is the man to pay close attention to and follow if you want a healthier, stronger and ultimately richer life experience. It has been an honor to know Dai as a coach, mentor and friend.” —KAYVAN

“The first few weeks were fun, with making small adjustments in my life and just making the commitment. I started looking at my calendar for the next day and seeing where I could fit in my 30 minutes. I quickly learned that I needed to go to bed earlier because my usual workout time is before the rest of the family is up, because that just works for me. A few weeks in, I started seeing the challenges coming up, and the outpouring of support from the community was amazing. So much encouragement from the team as well as personal support from Dai and Christie! This is a sustainable, lifelong fitness program. It is not just some fitness fad, it is the real deal.” —JENNIFER

“What a difference a year makes. Twelve months ago I was plagued with self-doubt. Fast forward to 2015 and I'm a new person thanks to the Whole Life Fitness program. In January, I would not have guessed that I could complete 90 days of WODs and not give up! I feel better, look better, and, most of all, I'm healthier—mentally and physically. I'm working harder but also enjoying the good things in life such as sharing a flavoured coffee with friends, sleeping in on the weekends, sampling desserts, and trying new foods—all guilt-free! I am loving myself back to life. Thank you, Dai!” —JILLIAN

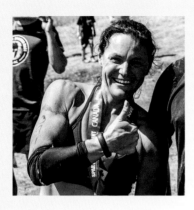

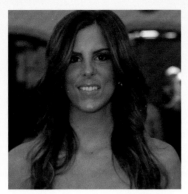

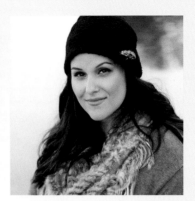

"What does the Whole Life Fitness Power 30 mean to me? It's a way to become mentally stronger and physically healthier. It's an overall life changer that can be done anywhere and anytime! You don't need weights, you don't need a gym, you just need to give YOURSELF two per cent of your day to create a whole new fantastic you! As they say, 'How can you care for others if you can't care for yourself?' So giving myself two per cent of the day so I can be a rock for others has made me much more than a rock—I'm a cliff now!" —AMANDA

"I am already seeing results in my arms, shoulders and legs. I know that sounds crazy because it's only week one, but even my husband notices! I feel stronger and I look more toned. More importantly, kids truly are little sponges! I walked into my son's room today and he was doing push-ups and counting. He scolded me when my will power failed and I went for a bag of potato chips. He likes to come to the track with me and watch me run. This is about more than me; it's about teaching my boys how to be healthy and take care of their bodies! Get healthy habits instilled in them now!" —MARIA

"In the first few weeks, I didn't notice many physical changes, but I was encouraged by how great I felt. I had increased energy levels, muscle strength and endurance, and a sense of well-being. At six weeks, changes became more visible even though my weight wasn't changing much; my arms and shoulders looked more toned, my belly got smaller and other people started to notice. Obviously weight isn't the most important thing, but it is so nice that I am fitting into my clothes better, some of which I haven't worn since before I had my baby 15 months ago." —PIA

It's Week 3—time to start ramping things up! You are starting to notice your increased energy, improved focus and overall sense of well-being. You are brimming with new ideas, rediscovering passions and looking forward to your daily 30-minute Whole Life Fitness Power 30 ritual. You are finding your flow and loving it!

This is also the week when you may doubt yourself and your commitment. Life gets busy, and that won't change, but remember why you started this program. If this happens to you, revisit your goals, or contribute to our online community at WholeLifeFitnessManifesto.com. There is a lot of power in connecting with others from the community. Believe you are capable, you are worthy, and you can do this.

Reflect back on Week 2 and write down one or two moments in which you surprised yourself. Maybe you did a double take at your own reflection, crushed a proposal for work, or weren't so on-edge with your family. Record your standout moments in your weekly journal.

A few things to shoot for this week:

1. Make a conscious effort to drink water every hour or so.
2. Truly challenge yourself to cut or limit yourself to three non-nutritional (treat) beverages over the week.
3. Enjoy at least one BAHG salad per day (big-ass healthy green salad).
4. Reach out and reconnect with one person with whom you have lost touch.
5. Continue being awesome!

EVERY DAY

- ✔ Drink two glasses of **water** upon waking.
- ✔ Complete a **warm-up** (optional, but recommended).
- ✔ **15-minute WOD** (workout of the day), as many rounds or repetitions as possible (AMRAP).
- ✔ Finish with a **cool-down** (optional, but recommended).
- ✔ Five minutes **meditation**: stillness, reflection and thankfulness.
- ✔ 10 minutes **personal development**. Feed your mind. Read, write, listen to inspiring ideas and information.

DAY-BY-DAY BREAKDOWN

When you finish one set of each exercise, start over until you reach the 15-minute mark. (And don't forget to record your score—how many rounds did you do?)

DAY 15
1. 20 seconds left-leg hopping
2. 20 seconds right-leg hopping
3. 20 seconds high-knee jogging on the spot
4. 20-second rest

DAY 16
1. 30 × jumping jacks
2. 20 × forward/back shuffle
3. 10 × skater lunges (side to side)

DAY 17
1. 15 × squats
2. 10 × push-ups
3. 20 × sit-ups

DAY 18
1. 20 mountain climbers (10 each leg)
2. 20 glute bridges

DAY 19
1. 20 × reverse swimmer (with a pause)
2. 30 seconds stationary sprints
3. 30-second rest

DAY 20
1. 10 push-ups (time yourself)
2. Rest for the same amount of time it took to complete the set of 10. Continue for 15 minutes.

DAY 21
1. 45–60-second plank
2. 45–60-second squat hold
3. 5 × burpees
4. 30-second rest

DAILY CHECKLIST

Use this checklist to help you organize your week.

Download a printable version from wholelifefitnessmanifesto.com/resources.

TO DO:	DRINK 2 TO 3L OF WATER	15 MINUTE WOD	5 MINUTES OF MINDFULNESS	10 MINUTES OF PERSONAL DEVELOPMENT	NO POP, NO ALCOHOL, NO PROBLEM	EAT A **BAHG** SALAD!	RECONNECT WITH A FRIEND
Sunday							
Monday							
Tuesday							
Wednesday							
Thursday							
Friday							
Saturday							

AND SO COMPLETES WEEK 3. KABOOM!

JOURNAL

Use this page for your victories, challenges, suggestions, comments and emotions.

Download a printable version from wholelifefitnessmanifesto.com/resources.

HOW DID IT GO?

» What changes have I noticed in my mood?
» How's my strength and stamina?
» How did I surprise myself this week?

Week 4 is here! Time for some extra fun as we ramp up our efforts and start to push our intensity a bit more. The daily Whole Life Fitness Power 30 ritual is becoming a lifelong habit—can you sense it? How good are you feeling? Pay attention to that sensation. Own it and be proud of it; you've worked hard to get here!

During Week 4, let's continue to build on everything we've done up to this point. A few things to shoot for this week:

1. Drink at least three litres of water each day.
2. Continue to avoid sugary beverages.
3. Aim to incorporate three whole-food, unprocessed meals with loads of greens per day.
4. Clean out your food cupboards and bring a donation to the local food bank.
5. Call someone who would appreciate and support your lifestyle change.

EVERY DAY

✔ Drink two glasses of **water** upon waking.

✔ Complete a **warm-up** (optional, but recommended).

✔ **15-minute WOD** (workout of the day), as many rounds or repetitions as possible (AMRAP).

✔ Finish with a **cool-down** (optional, but recommended).

✔ Five minutes **meditation**: stillness, reflection and thankfulness.

✔ 10 minutes **personal development**. Feed your mind. Read, write, listen to inspiring ideas and information.

DAY-BY-DAY BREAKDOWN

When you finish one set of each exercise, start over until you reach the 15-minute mark. (And don't forget to record your score—how many rounds did you do?)

DAY 22
1. 20 × alternating lunges (10 per leg)
2. 10 × chair/bench step-ups

DAY 23
1. 5 × push-ups
2. 10 × sit-ups
3. 15 × squats

DAY 24
1. Part One: 7-minute AMRAP
   - 10 × step-ups
   - 15 × glute-bridges
   One-minute rest
2. Part Two: 7-minute AMRAP
   - 30-second plank
   - 30 seconds air skips

DAY 25
1. 5 × caterpillar stretches
2. 10 × jumping jacks
3. 15 × lateral hops

DAY 26
1. 5 × push-ups
2. 10 × sit-ups
3. 15 × reverse swimmers (alternating)

DAY 27
1. 15 minutes of walking, talking and smiling (if you're doing this indoors, consider dancing your heart out—seriously get down and boogie!). Enjoy your surroundings, be silly, have fun!

DAY 28
1. WOD: 100 burpees (yeah, burpees!) for time or 15 minutes, whichever comes first. Just keep moving, no matter the pace (and of course keep smiling as you curse my name under your breath—LOL!)

DAILY CHECKLIST

Use this checklist to help you organize your week.

Download a printable version from wholelifefitnessmanifesto.com/resources.

TO DO:	DRINK 3L OF WATER	15 MINUTE WOD	5 MINUTES OF MINDFULNESS	10 MINUTES OF PERSONAL DEVELOPMENT	NO POP, NO ALCOHOL, NO PROBLEM	THREE HEALTHY MEALS A DAY	SHARE MY AWESOMENESS WITH FRIENDS
Sunday							
Monday							
Tuesday							
Wednesday							
Thursday							
Friday							
Saturday							

AND SO COMPLETES WEEK 4.
... YOU MADE IT, HECK YES! #JUSTDIDIT

JOURNAL

Use this page for your victories, challenges, suggestions, comments and emotions.

Download a printable version from wholelifefitnessmanifesto.com/resources.

HOW DID IT GO?

» What changes am I noticing in my body shape?

» How am I feeling about my own abilities?

» How are the people who love me responding to the changes in me?

See how far you've come?

Congratulations, you made it!

To get a clear picture of how your fitness has improved, it's time to retake the baseline fitness test (on page 135). Also, take your measurements, along with new photos, and compare them to the ones you took at the beginning of the program. Pretty awesome!

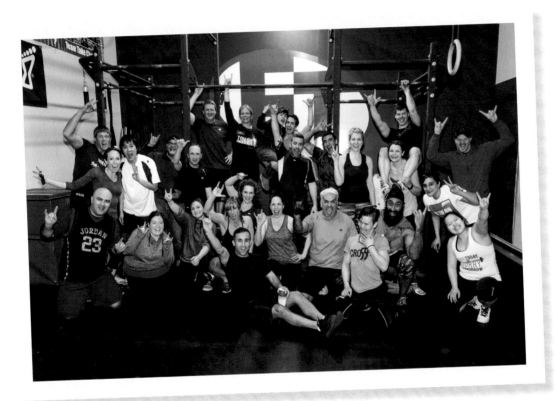

#JUSTDIDIT

DONE!

FINAL CHECKLIST ✔

RE-TAKE BASELINE FITNESS TEST	
RE-TAKE MEASUREMENTS	
RE-TAKE PHOTOS	
LOOK IN THE MIRROR AND SAY "I'M AWESOME!"	
PAY IT FORWARD—WHO DO YOU KNOW THAT COULD BENEFIT FROM A HEALTHY CHANGE?	
ASK YOURSELF: "WHAT'S NEXT FOR MY HEALTH AND WELLNESS GOALS?"	

Now that you've finished the first four weeks, it's time to reset and reevaluate your goals. You might go for a second phase of the Whole Life Fitness Power 30 program, and see how different it feels the next time around. Just think of the rock-solid foundation you've already built! Alternatively, you might choose to design your own workouts, following similar principles. Pick and mix from the exercises list on page 158, and slot them into the chart on page 159. Or, for those who like to have a plan to follow, check out these fun options.

Basic Pick-n-Mix

Choose one lower body movement, one upper body movement and one core movement per day. Set the amount of reps per round, or amount of time spent doing each movement per round. See how many rounds or reps you can complete in 15 minutes.

Example:

- 10 × squats,
- 10 × push-ups,
- 30 seconds of sit-ups per 15 minute AMRAP (as many reps or rounds as possible)

The "Hot, Bold or Spicy" Challenge

Create your own 15-minute workouts on a two-days-on, one-day-off schedule for 30 days. Choose three to five exercises from the list, then decide on a number of reps (5, 10, 15) or time (15, 30 or 45 seconds). Be sure to choose at least one upper body, one lower body and one core movement, e.g., push-ups, squats and plank. Mix it up! Don't be afraid to experiment. And most importantly, HAVE FUN!

Example:

- Hot: 5 × push-ups, 5 × squats, 15-second plank for 15 minutes. How many rounds can I do?
- Bold: 10 × push-ups, 10 × squats, 30-second plank. Repeat for 15 minutes.
- Spicy: 15 × push-ups, 15 × squats, 45-second plank. Repeat for 15 minutes.

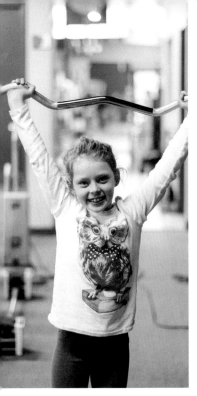
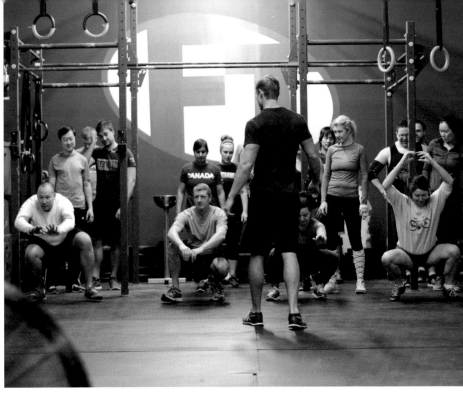
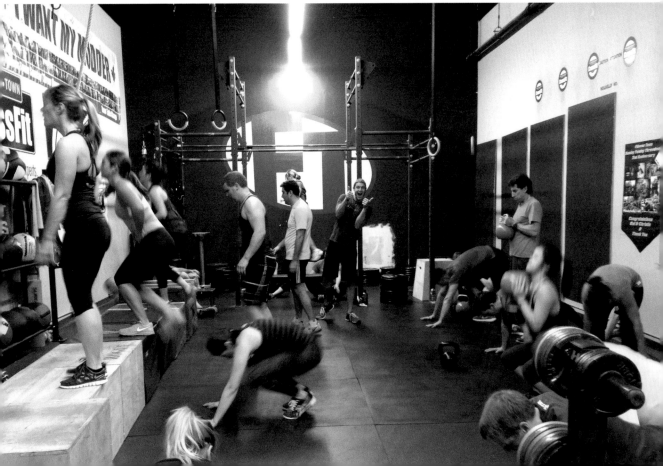

PICK-N-MIX EXERCISES LIST

UPPER BODY	LOWER BODY	CORE
Push-up or Variation	Squat	Sit-ups
Burpee	Step-up	Plank — Elbow
Caterpillar Stretch	Lunge — Forward	*Plebs Plank
Dips	Lunge — Reverse	*Hollow Rock
Mountain Climbers	Air Skips	Bicycle
*Diamond Push-up	Glute Bridge	Butterfly Situp
*Elevated Feet Push-up	High-knee jog	Side Plank
*Lateral Plank Walk	Jumping Jacks	Plank Up / Plank Down
*Reverse Plank Bridge	*Lunge Twist	Crunch
*Superman	Squat Jump	Seated Twist
*Good Mornings	Skater Lunge	
*Push-up w/ One Arm Reach	Leg Hops	
Reverse Swimmers	Lateral Hops	
*Handstand Hold	*Sumo Squat	
*Arm Circles	*Wide Squat w/Calf Raise	
*Pull-up (if you have a pull-up bar)	*Calf Raises	
*Jumping Pull-ups	*Squat Reach	
*Air Boxing	*Squat with Back Kick	
	Wall Sit	
	Feet Shuffle	
	*Squat with Side Leg Raise	
	*Donkey Kicks	

* Find a description of this movement at www.WholeLifeFitnessManifesto.com/exercises

BODY SECTION	CHOOSE YOUR OWN MOVEMENT!	CHOOSE HOW MANY REPS PER ROUND, OR HOW MUCH TIME IN SECONDS PER ROUND	RESULTS: HOW MANY ROUNDS DID YOU DO IN 15 MINUTES?
Day One			
Upper Body			
Lower Body			
Core			
Day Two			
Upper Body			
Lower Body			
Core			
Day Three			
Upper Body			
Lower Body			
Core			
Day Four			
Upper Body			
Lower Body			
Core			
Day Five			
Upper Body			
Lower Body			
Core			
Day Six			
Upper Body			
Lower Body			
Core			
Day Seven			
Upper Body			
Lower Body			
Core			

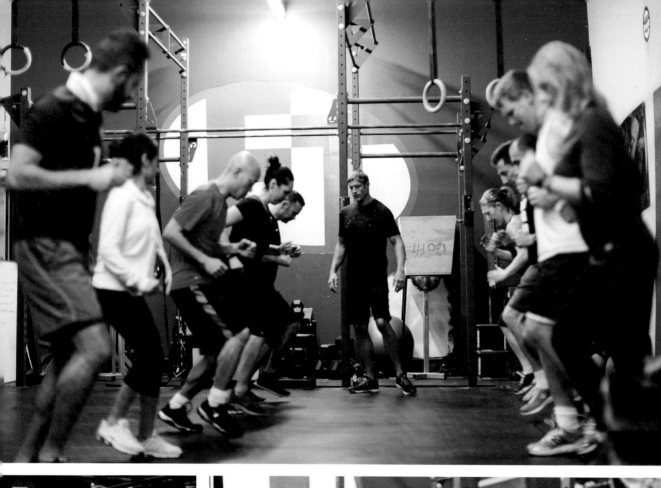

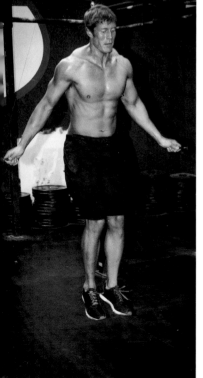

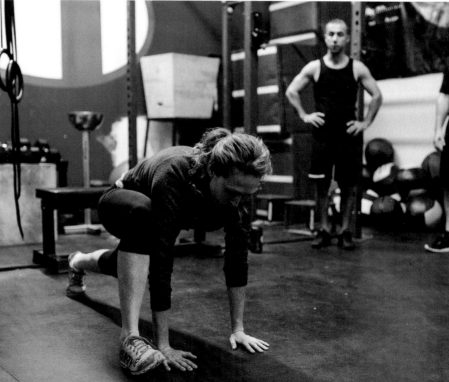

The joy of running is that it can be done literally anywhere. Lace up your sneakers, complete a quick warm-up, and off you go. However, there is nothing like adding a little variety to your run to keep you even more motivated. Turn the page for an arsenal of running-based exercise routines to keep you moving forward.

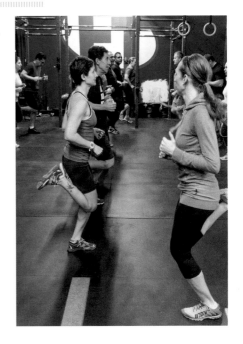

Example Workout:

Hot (5 rounds):

* 1 minute of running
* 1 minute of squats

Bold (7 rounds):

* 1 minute of running
* 1 minute of squats

Spicy (10 rounds):

* 1 minute of running
* 1 minute of squats

Go to www.WholeLifeFitnessManifesto.com to check out recently added workouts and other fitness plans to motivate you.

RUNNING WORKOUTS

Run 1.6 km (1 mile). Stop every one minute to complete 10 squats, 10 push-ups and 10 sit-ups

10 rounds for time:
- 10 × burpees, 100-metre sprint, OR
- 10 × push-ups, 100-metre sprint

10 sets of 100-metre sprint (rest for length of time it took you to complete the previous sprint)

10 × 50-metre sprint (rest for two minutes between sprints)

Four rounds for time: 20 × sit-ups, 20 × push-ups, 400-metre run

Three rounds for time: Run 0.8 km (0.5 miles), 50 x squats

Three rounds for time: 400-metre run, 30 x squats

Five rounds: 200-metre sprint (rest for length of time it took you to complete the previous sprint)

Three rounds: 50 × sit-ups, 400-metre run, sprint or walk.

Five 400-metre sprints (rest for the length of time it took you to complete the previous sprint)

Run 1.6 km (1 mile), completing 10 × push-ups every one minute

Run 1.6 km (1 mile) for time

Run 1.6 km (1 mile), completing 100 × squats at midpoint, for time

Run 1.6 km (1 mile), completing 30 × lunges every one minute

Run 1.6 km (1 mile), 50 × squats for time

Run 1.6 km (1 mile), completing 20 × squats every one minute

Five rounds: Run one minute, squats for one minute

RUNNING WORKOUTS

Three rounds: 200-metre run, 50 × squats

Four rounds: 400-metre run, 50 × squats

Three rounds for time: 400-metre run, 30 × air squats, then a 30-second handstand hold

Five rounds: Run with high knees for 15 seconds, drop into a push-up, run with high knees for 15 more seconds.

10 rounds: 100-metre sprint, 100-metre walk

Eight rounds: 100-metre sprint, 30 × squats

Three rounds: 200-metre spring, 25 × push-ups

10 rounds: 50-metre sprint, 10 × push-ups

10 rounds for time: 100-metre sprint, 20 × squats

Record your scores and try the same workout in 30 days.

Go to www.WholeLifeFitnessManifesto.com to check out recently added workouts and other fitness plans to motivate you.

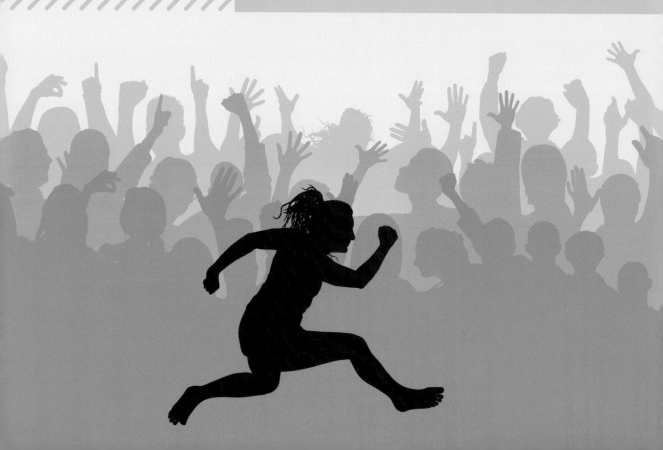

HEALTHY FOR
THE LONG HAUL
CHAPTER 9

NOW THAT YOU KNOW HEALTH is the foundation from which everything else flourishes, you're all set to create a life of awesomeness! It's my hope that the *Whole Life Fitness Manifesto* has ignited your passion and got you raring to go.

Look back on the difficulties you've faced with earlier attempts to become healthier and happier. You've probably already learned that there are no instant fixes when it comes to fitness and health, but I hope I've provided you with some healthy habits that you are willing to put into action.

Our futures are largely determined by the choices and actions we make today. Thankfully, it's never too late to make changes that will put us on a better trajectory. Can you sense the possibilities?

We all know that life can get in the way of even the most established routines. Most of us will need to work around recovery from an illness or injury at some point. Don't feel bad about slowing down a little to let yourself heal—that's what you're supposed to do! But even if you can't work out quite as hard or use every muscle group in the same way, it's important to keep the habit going strong. As long as you're doing *something* to move your body, with purpose and intent, for 15 minutes a day and, ideally, refuelling your mind through meditation and personal development, then I'm happy. Just don't give up.

It's perfectly okay to switch things up and add a little variety when inspiration strikes! Who knows what new activity you might discover in the future; Maybe you'll develop a love of running, yoga or dance. It's great to change up your workout routine to do more of what you enjoy most.

We only get one life, so why not make the most of it and experience all that we can? Push yourself to try new experiences. Your choices are endless! Say *HECK YES!*

"Don't count the days, make the days count."
—MUHAMMAD ALI

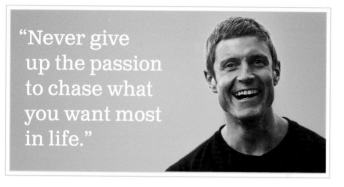

"Never give up the passion to chase what you want most in life."

to new opportunities, knowing that you have the health and fitness, along with the confidence in yourself, to enjoy new adventures, whatever they may be. With the *Whole Life Fitness Manifesto*, my aim is to encourage you to pursue as full a life as possible; a life that you can look back on without regrets.

Remember that we don't have to settle for average. I'm all for appreciating what we have—our families, our homes, our jobs—but it's important to strive to be better every day, because that's how we grow. My hope is that the Whole Life Fitness Power 30 will inject a bit of greatness into your day, that it will make you *feel* great, and that it will propel you to shoot for so much more, aiming a little higher in everything you do.

In addition, remember that there are major benefits to taking time out of every day for a few minutes of mindful meditation. By establishing a *Whole Life Fitness* ritual that tones your mind and spirit as well as your body, you're setting yourself up to be healthy for the long haul. And when that happens, not only will you conquer your personal fitness goals, you'll also empower others to take control of their health. Can I get a big hoorah for that? HOO-RAH!

> "Whatever you can do, or dream you can, begin it. Boldness has genius, power, and magic in it."
>
> —GOETHE

And of course, life isn't just about you or me—it's about *us*. We need each other. The *Whole Life Fitness Manifesto* is based on a sense of community. Each participant has the capacity to hold each other accountable, but also to support each other, to have fun and bring joy to our tribe members. We can always count on our tribe to pick us up when we're down, and encourage us to follow through on our personal commitments and goals, because they have our best interests in mind. Just as Michelangelo saw his masterpiece, *David*, within a block of marble, our tribe can also see the potential in each of us. Through emotional support, unconditional friendship and accountability, we draw the masterpiece from within each other.

My friend, I want to thank you for allowing me the opportunity to enter your life, and for reading this book. It's my hope that the narrative doesn't end here. Reach out to me and the *Whole Life Fitness Manifesto* community online (www.WholeLifeFitnessManifesto.com) so we can support one another, share in our ups and downs, bring a life of awesomeness to all those we meet, and ultimately, carry one another to a new pinnacle of purpose, passion and drive.

The *Whole Life Fitness Manifesto* community doesn't judge, point fingers or lay blame. In joining us online you open yourself up to a community of like-minded people wanting very similar things. It's also where I share the latest information, workouts, tips and reviews to help you cut through all the noise relating to health, fitness, wellness and lifestyle, and I will continue to do so for as long as I can.

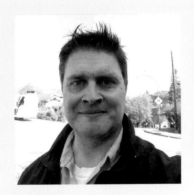

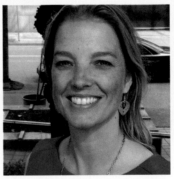

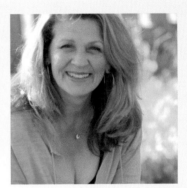

" I recently completed the Whole Life Fitness Power 30, and wow, what an experience! Dai's guidance was a blast. He's a great teacher and motivator, and the information in the program has been easy to understand and integrate into everyday life."

—MARK

" Personally, I think it's all about community, making new friends and seeing results, and Dai has done that. I'm stronger, leaner and happier, and I walk around with more self-confidence! Dai's energy and happiness is contagious and he's making our community (and soon the world) a better place!"

—CAROLINE

" The Whole Life Fitness Power 30 is an amazing journey. I wanted to learn how to be accountable, consistent and healthier. I also wanted tools to become a better leader and help others, and this gave me so much more. I love myself more than I ever have before."—LISA

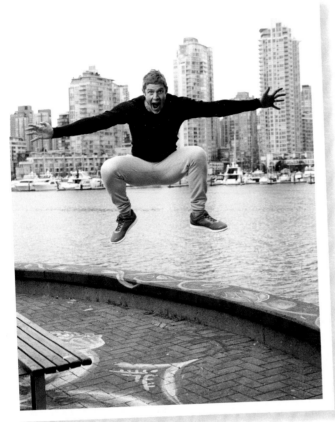

What does it mean to live a life of no regrets, of optimized mind, body and spirit? One word comes to my mind—FUN! I strive to enjoy every waking moment, appreciating the friendships I form and the family I'm raising, as well as helping others in my tribe experience the incredible, epic journey of life. That's my *WHY*.

We are companions on this journey to greatness, and it's the trip of a lifetime. You might be working out on your own, but you're never alone. I'm happy and honoured to be taking the first step of a long, fulfilling journey with you today. Never stop honouring your *why*. Keep your vision at the front of your mind and let it be the filter through which you look at your life choices from now on. The limitations that you had yesterday don't apply today, and if you think that's amazing, just wait to see what tomorrow brings.

NOTES

CHAPTER ONE

9.   *and socially stimulated* Maia Szalavitz, "Touching Empathy," *Psychology Today* (March 1, 2010), https://www.psychologytoday.com/blog/born-love/201003/touching-empathy (Accessed August 6, 2015).

11. *miracles in and of themselves* Charles Q. Choi, "'Invisible Gorilla' Test Shows How Little We Notice," *Live Science* (July 11, 2010), http://www.livescience.com/6727-invisible-gorilla-test-shows-notice.html (Accessed July 12, 2015).

11. *Take The Invisible Gorilla* Charles Q. Choi, "'Invisible Gorilla' Test Shows How Little We Notice," *Live Science* (July 11, 2010), http://www.livescience.com/6727-invisible-gorilla-test-shows-notice.html (Accessed August 5, 2015).

12. *the secrets to a long life* Dan Buettner, *The Blue Zones: 9 Lessons for Living Longer from the People Who've Lived the Longest*, Second edition, National Geographic Society (November 6, 2012).

12. *just for the fun of it!* "Piano Stairs," *TheFunTheory.com* (2009), http://www.thefuntheory.com/piano-staircase (Accessed August 5, 2015).

12. *performed 30 squats* Andrew Bender, "Moscow Subway Station Lets Passengers Pay Fare in Squats," *Forbes* (November 14, 2013), http://www.forbes.com/sites/andrewbender/2013/11/14/moscow-subway-station-lets-passengers-pay-fare-in-squats/ (Accessed August 5, 2015).

16. *daily in the 1970s* Caitlin Johnson, "Cutting Through Advertising Clutter," *CBS News* (September 17, 2006), http://www.cbsnews.com/news/cutting-through-advertising-clutter/ (Accessed August 5, 2015).

CHAPTER TWO

21. *the secrets to a long life* Dan Buettner, *The Blue Zones: 9 Lessons for Living Longer from the People Who've Lived the Longest*, Second edition, National Geographic Society (November 6, 2012). *risk factor for global mortality* World Health Organization (blog), "Health Topics: Physical Activity," http://www.who.int/topics/physical_activity/en/ (Accessed August 19, 2015).

21. *physical inactivity is now identified* World Health Organization, Global Recommendations on Physical Activity for Health (Geneva: WHO Press, 2010)

CHAPTER THREE

39. *diabetes, and heart disease* Darren E.R. Warburton, Crystal Whitney Nicol, Shannon S.D. Bredin, "Health benefits of physical activity: the evidence," US National Library of Medicine

National Institutes of Health, 174(6): 801-809 (March 14, 2006), http://www.ncbi.nlm.nih.gov/pmc/articles/PMC1402378/ (Accessed August 6, 2015).

39.   *a medical diagnosis* Dr. I-Min Lee, Eric J. Shiroma, Felipe Lobelo, Pekka Puska, Steven N. Blair, Peter T. Katzmarzyk, "Effects of physical inactivity on major non-communicable diseases worldwide: an analysis of burden of disease and life expectancy," The Lancet, Volume 380, No. 9838 (July 18, 2012), http://www.thelancet.com/journals/lancet/article/PIIS0140-6736(12)61031-9/abstract (Accessed August 6, 2015).

39.   *our bodies are designed to move* Charles E. Matthews, Kong Y. Chen, Patty S. Freedson, Maciej S. Buchowski, Bettina M. Beech, Russell R. Pate, Richard P. Troiano, "Amount of Time Spent in Sedentary Behaviors in the United States, 2003-2004," American Journal of Epidemiology, 167 (7): 875-881 (December 11, 2007), http://aje.oxfordjournals.org/content/167/7/875.full (Accessed August 5, 2015).

39.   *men who sit more* A.V. Patel, L. Bernstein, A. Deka, H.S. Feigelson, P.T. Campbell, S.M. Gapstur, G.A. Colditz, M.J. Thun, "Leisure Time Spent Sitting in Relation to Total Mortality in a Prospective Cohort of US Adults," US National Library of Medicine National Institutes of Health, 172 (4): 419-29 (August 15, 2010), http://www.ncbi.nlm.nih.gov/pubmed/20650954 (Accessed August 5, 2015).

40.   *since the 1960s* Timothy S. Church, Diana M. Thomas, Catrine Tudor-Locke, Peter T. Katzmarzyk, Conrad P. Earnest, Ruben Q. Rodarte, Corby K. Martin, Steven N. Blair, Claude Bouchard, "Trends over 5 Decades in U.S. Occupation-Related Physical Activity and Their Associations with Obesity," *PLoS ONE* (May 25, 2011), http://journals.plos.org/plosone/article?id=10.1371/journal.pone.0019657 (Accessed August 5, 2015).

40.   *jobs that are largely inactive!* "The Price of Inactivity," *American Heart Association* (July 31, 2015), http://www.heart.org/HEARTORG/GettingHealthy/PhysicalActivity/FitnessBasics/The-Price-of-Inactivity_UCM_307974_Article.jsp (Accessed August 5, 2015).

40.   *than they did in the 1960s.* Timothy S. Church, Diana M. Thomas, Catrine Tudor-Locke, Peter T. Katzmarzyk, Conrad P. Earnest, Ruben Q. Rodarte, Corby K. Martin, Steven N. Blair, Claude Bouchard, "Trends over 5 Decades in U.S. Occupation-Related Physical Activity and Their Associations with Obesity," *PLoS ONE* (May 25, 2011), http://journals.plos.org/plosone/article?id=10.1371/journal.pone.0019657 (Accessed August 5, 2015).

40.   *2,100 calories per day.* Dr. Stephan Guyenet, "The American Diet." TEDX video, 16:35 (Posted February 6, 2012), http://tedxtalks.ted.com/video/TEDxHarvardLaw-Stephan-Guyene-2 (Accessed August 19, 2015).

40.   *It's stress* Full Report: Towers Watson/NBGH 2013/2014 Employer Survey on Purchasing Value in Health Care (May 2014), http://www.towerswatson.com/en/Insights/IC-Types/Survey-Research-Results/2014/05/full-report-towers-watson-nbgh-2013-2014-employer-survey-on-purchasing-value-in-health-care (Accessed August 19, 2015).

40.   *$12.8 billion per year!* Darrell J. Gaskin, Ph.D. and Patrick Richard, Ph.D., M.A., "Relieving Pain in America: A Blueprint for Transforming Prevention, Care, Education, and Research," *National Center for Biotechnology Information* (2011), http://www.ncbi.nlm.nih.gov/books/NBK92521/ (Accessed August 19, 2015).

40.   *in lost productivity* 2011 Dan Witters and Sangeeta Agrawal, "Unhealthy U.S. Workers' Absenteeism Costs $153 Billion," *Gallup* (October 17, 2011), http://www.gallup.com/poll/150026/unhealthy-workers-absenteeism-costs-153-billion.aspx (Accessed August 19, 2015).

40.   *corporate wellness programs?* "Companies Are Spending More on Corporate Wellness Programs but Employees Are Leaving Millions on the Table," *Business Wire* (March 26, 2015), http://www

.businesswire.com/news/home/20150326005585/en/Companies-Spending-Corporate-Wellness-Programs-Employees-Leaving#.VYNx2_lVhBc (Accessed August 5, 2015).

42. *get a BHAG!* Jim Collins, Jerry I. Porras, *Built to Last: Successful Habits of Visionary Companies*, Harper Collins (June 24, 2004).

CHAPTER FOUR
||||||||||||||||||||||||||||||||||||||||||||||||||||||||

47. *behaviours such as sitting* Charles E. Matthews, Kong Y. Chen, Patty S. Freedson, Maciej S. Buchowski, Bettina M. Beech, Russell R. Pate, Richard P. Troiano, "Amount of Time Spent in Sedentary Behaviors in the United States, 2003-2004," *American Journal of Epidemiology*, 167 (7): 875-881 (December 11, 2007), http://aje.oxfordjournals.org/content/167/7/875.full (Accessed August 5, 2015).

47. *inactivity, in particular, sitting* A.V. Patel, L. Bernstein, A. Deka, H.S. Feigelson, P.T. Campbell, S.M. Gapstur, G.A. Colditz, M.J. Thun, "Leisure Time Spent Sitting in Relation to Total Mortality in a Prospective Cohort of US Adults," *US National Library of Medicine National Institutes of Health*, 172 (4): 419-29 (August 15, 2010), http://www.ncbi.nlm.nih.gov/pubmed/20650954 (Accessed August 5, 2015).

48. *to the tube* Norman Herr, PhD, "Television & Health," *Internet Resources to Accompany The Sourcebook for Teaching Science*, http://www.csun.edu/science/health/docs/tv&health.html (Accessed August 5, 2015).

48. *viewing a week!* Michael Oliveira, "TV Viewership: Canadians Watch 30 Hours Of TV A Week, And Spend More Time Online," *Huffington Post* (April 25, 2013), http://www.huffingtonpost.ca/2013/04/25/tv-viewership-canada-online_n_3156176.html (Accessed August 5, 2015).

48. *3.5 minutes per week!* Martin Turcotte, "Time spent with family during a typical workday, 1986 to 2005," *Canadian Social Trends, Statistics Canada Catalogue* http://www.statcan.gc.ca/pub/11-008-x/2006007/9574-eng.htm (Accessed August 19, 2015).

48. *insufficiently physically active.* World Health Organization (blog), "Media Centre: Physical Activity Fact Sheet," http://www.who.int/mediacentre/factsheets/fs385/en/ (Accessed August 5, 2015).

53. *7 hours and 48 minutes* Report Card on Physical Activity for Children and Youth, Active Healthy Kids Canada (2012) http://www.participaction.com/wp-content/uploads/2015/03/AHKC-2012-Report-Card-Short-Form-FINAL.pdf (Accessed August 5, 2015).

53. *parents spend at work!* "Learn the Facts," ParticipACTION (2013), http://www.participaction.com/make-room-for-play-2/learn-the-facts/ (Accessed August 6, 2015).

CHAPTER FIVE
||||||||||||||||||||||||||||||||||||||||||||||||||||||||

59. *effectively replace painkillers* P. la Cour, M. Petersen, "Effects of mindfulness meditation on chronic pain: a randomized controlled trial," *US National Library of Medicine National Institutes of Health*, (4): 641-52 (April 16, 2015), http://www.ncbi.nlm.nih.gov/pubmed/25376753 (Accessed August 5, 2015).

60. *issues and fibromyalgia* Steven D. Ehrlich, NMD, "Mind-body medicine," *University of Maryland Medical Center* (October 2, 2011), http://umm.edu/health/medical/altmed/treatment/mindbody-medicine (Accessed August 5, 2015).

60. *harder to think clearly* "Alcohol," *Young Men's Health* (May 14, 2014), http://www.youngmenshealthsite.org/alcohol_effects_on_brain_and_body.html (Accessed August 5, 2015).

61.   *developing depression* A. Sanchez-Villegas, E. Toledo, J. de Irala, M. Ruiz-Canela, J. Pla-Vidal, M.A. Martinez-Gonzalez, "Fast-food and commercial baked goods consumption and the risk of depression," *US National Library of Medicine National Institutes of Health* (3): 424-32 (March 15, 2012), http://www.ncbi.nlm.nih.gov/pubmed/21835082 (Accessed August 5, 2015).

61.   *another state of being* Kendra Cherry, "What Is Flow? Understanding the Psychology of Flow," *About.com*, http://psychology.about.com/od/PositivePsychology/a/flow.htm (Accessed August 5, 2015).

61.   *Dr. Mihaly Csikszentmihalyi* Kendra Cherry, "What Is Flow? Understanding the Psychology of Flow," *About.com*, http://psychology.about.com/od/PositivePsychology/a/flow.htm (Accessed August 5, 2015).

63.   *changing unproductive habits* Diane Toroian Keaggy, "Breaking down stress: Mindfulness, breathing and yoga can beat back stress' side effects," *Washington University in St. Louis* (December 10, 2013), http://news.wustl.edu/news/Pages/26265.aspx (Accessed August 5, 2015).

65.   *the results we're after* Ed Halliwell, "Meditate with Intention, Not Goals," *Mindful*, (October 15, 2014), http://www.mindful.org/meditate-with-intention-not-goals/ (Accessed August 5, 2015).

67.   *information more slowly* Ozge Ozkaya, "Calming the mind," *Free Meditation* (September 10, 2009), http://www.freemeditation.com/articles/2009/09/10/calming-the-mind/ (Accessed August 5, 2015).

67.   *into "sleep mode" during meditation.* Rebecca Gladding, "This Is Your Brain on Meditation," *Psychology Today* (May 22, 2013), https://www.psychologytoday.com/blog/use-your-mind-change-your-brain/201305/is-your-brain-meditation (Accessed August 5, 2015).

67.   *slows down during meditation* Rebecca Gladding, "This Is Your Brain on Meditation," *Psychology Today* (May 22, 2013), https://www.psychologytoday.com/blog/use-your-mind-change-your-brain/201305/is-your-brain-meditation (Accessed August 5, 2015).

67.   *areas of the brain* Britta K. Holzel, James Carmody, Mark Vangel, Christina Congleton, Sita M. Yerramsetti, Tim Gard, Sara W. Lazar, "Mindfulness practice leads to increases in regional brain gray matter density," *US National Library of Medicine National Institutes of Health* (November 10, 2010), http://www.ncbi.nlm.nih.gov/pmc/articles/PMC3004979/ (Accessed August 5, 2015).

67.   *silence and peace* Deepak Chopra, M.D., "7 Myths of Meditation," *Chopra Centered Lifestyle*, http://www.chopra.com/ccl/7-myths-of-meditation (Accessed August 5, 2015).

71.   *choice, and discipline* James C. Collins, "GoodReads Quotable Quote," http://www.goodreads.com/quotes/651191-greatness-is-not-a-function-of-circumstance-greatness-it-turns (Accessed August 5, 2015).

CHAPTER SIX

74.   *my vision boards* Jack Canfield, "How to Create an Empowering Vision Board," *Jack Canfield: Maximizing Your Potential* (December 3, 2014), http://jackcanfield.com/how-to-create-an-empowering-vision-book/ (Accessed August 5, 2015).

76.   *blood-sugar levels* "What is the Glycemic Index?" The World's Healthiest Foods (2015), http://www.whfoods.com/genpage.php?tname=faq&dbid=32 (Accessed August 6, 2015).

76.   *stroke, depression and more* Jane Higdon, Victoria J. Drake, Simin Liu, "Glycemic Index and Glycemic Load," Linus Pauling Institute Micronutrient Information Center (February, 2009), http://lpi.oregonstate.edu/mic/food-beverages/glycemic-index-glycemic-load (Accessed August 6, 2015).

77. *Dietary Guidelines*, Office of Disease Prevention and Health Promotion, (2010), http://health.gov/dietaryguidelines/ (Accessed August 6, 2015).

80. *just one drink!* "Sugar 101," American Heart Association (November 19, 2014), http://www.heart.org/HEARTORG/GettingHealthy/NutritionCenter/HealthyEating/Sugar-101_UCM_306024_Article.jsp (Accessed August 6, 2015).

81. *and reduce inflammation* Kathy Smart, *Live The Smart Way: Gluten Free Cookbook* (Toronto: Dundurn, 2011).

84. *revelry, and celebration?* P. Rozin, M. Ashmore, M. Markwith, "Lay American conceptions of nutrition: dose insensitivity, categorical thinking, contagion, and the monotonic mind," *US National Library of Medicine National Institutes of Health* (6): 438-47 (November 15, 1996), http://www.ncbi.nlm.nih.gov/pubmed/8973924 (Accessed August 5, 2015).

CHAPTER EIGHT

131. *Some say it takes* 21 *days* Jeremy Dean, *Making Habits, Breaking Habits: Why We Do Things, Why We Don't*, and How to Make Any Change Stick (Philadelphia: Da Capo Press, 2013).

131. *it might take longer* Phillippa Lally, Cornelia H. M. van Jaarsveld, Henry W.W. Potts, Jane Wardle, "How are habits formed: Modelling habit formation in the real world," European Journal of Social Psychology, Vol. 40 Issue 6 (July 16, 2009), http://onlinelibrary.wiley.com/doi/10.1002/ejsp.674/abstract (Accessed August 6, 2015).

131. *In* 2009 *Phillippa Lally* Phillippa Lally, Cornelia H. M. van Jaarsveld, Henry W.W. Potts, Jane Wardle, "How are habits formed: Modelling habit formation in the real world," European Journal of Social Psychology, Vol. 40 Issue 6 (July 16, 2009), http://onlinelibrary.wiley.com/doi/10.1002/ejsp.674/abstract (Accessed August 6, 2015).

134. 10 *components of physical fitness*, Jim Crawley, CrossFit (May 30, 2003), http://www.crossfit.com/mt-archive2/000056.html (Accessed August 6, 2015).

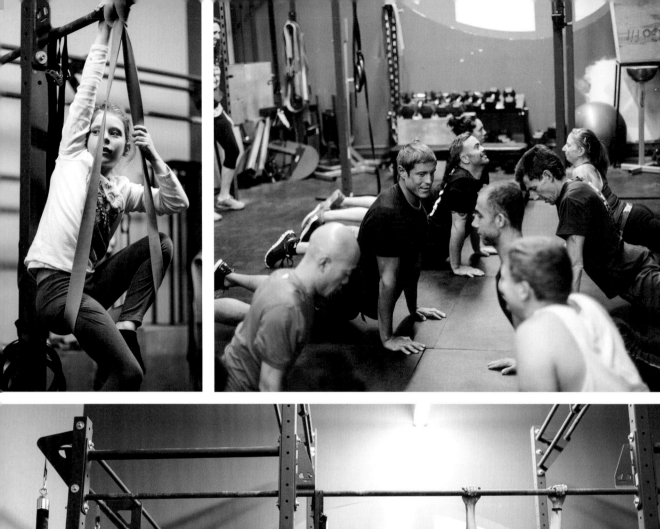
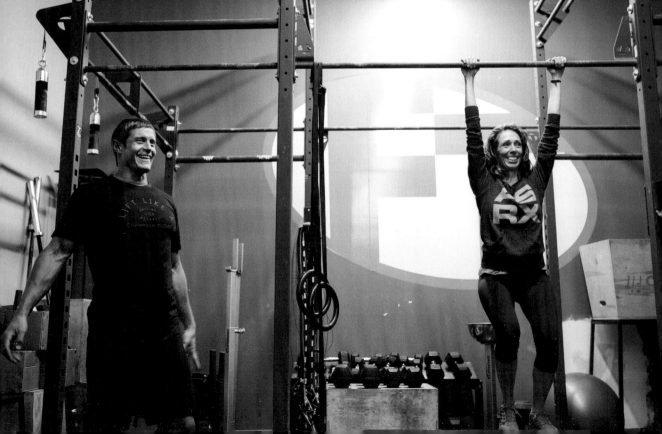

INDEX

children
    interactions with, 9, 48
    motivation from, 8, 19, 35
    physical activity trends of, 21, 53
    role-modelling for, 7
Chopra, Deepak, 67
Collins, Jim, 42, 71
commitments to self, 13–14, 17, 38–39,
        48–49, 57, 165–166
cool-down routines, 130
core moves
    Bicycle, 127
    Butterfly Sit-up, 118
    Caterpillar Stretch, 96–97
    Crunch, 98
    Feet Shuffle (alternating), 100
    Glute Bridge, 101
    High-Knee Jogging (on the
        spot), 102
    Planks, 112–114
    Reverse Swimmer, 117
    Seated Twist, 126
corpse pose, 16–17
CrossFit, 50–52
Crunch, 98
Csikszentmihalyi, Mihaly, 61

D

daily checklists, 138, 140, 142, 148, 152
diet
    Dai Manuel's story, 73–75
    enjoyment of, 79–80, 83–85
    guidelines and advice, 76, 78, 82–83
    portion sizing, 78, 79

and travel, 38
    see also foods
dining tips, 84
Dips (chair), 99

E

eating habits
    and longevity, 12
    tracking, 75
    see also diet
empathy, 9
energy
    increases in, 7, 15, 28, 33
    levels and glycemic index, 76
    see also mental energy
equipment, 86–87
excuses, overcoming, 13–14, 35–39, 41,
        44–45
exercise
    basic moves illustrated, 90–127
    in everyday functioning, 6
    the Good, Bad, and Ugly, 28
    and nutrition, 78–79
    Pick-n-Mix list, 158
    warm-up and cool-down routines,
        130
    see also running

F

faith
    Dai Manuel's story, 25–26
    and longevity, 12
    and well-being, 10–11

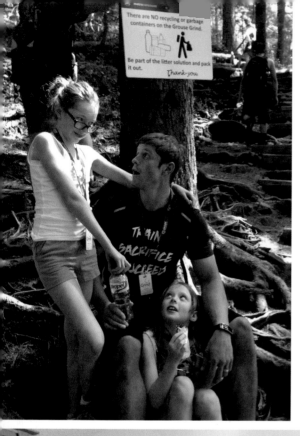

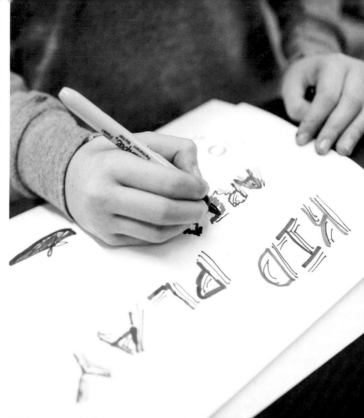

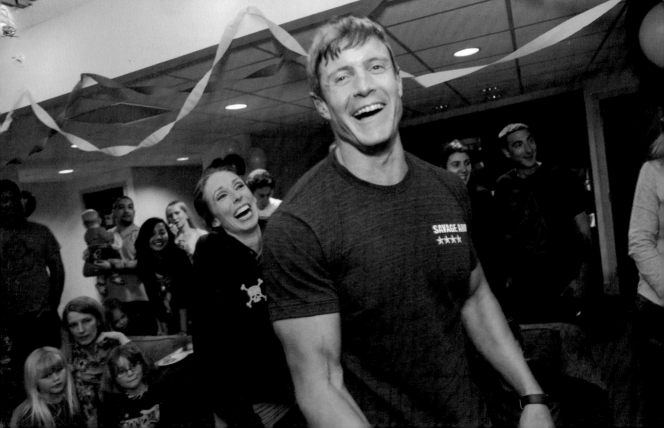

ACKNOWLEDGMENTS

LIFE IS LIKE A BURPEE. It offers momentary bouts of discomfort and adversity, along with opportunities to grow and improve. To those who embrace these challenges, live life to the fullest, and never settle for "good enough," this book is for you. You inspire me and keep me pressing forward no matter what obstacles stand in my way.

To my fabulous wife with the *tinge-of-ginge*, Christie, without whom I would be half the man I am today, I cannot thank you enough for your unconditional friendship and love. I've never been more excited to show you my gratitude each day for the rest of our lives… and of course, to chase the sun and live our adventures together. I love you dearly.

To my daughters, Chardonae and Brielyn, you are my *raison d'etre*. My "why" shifted drastically the day I became a father. You hold me accountable to be the best man, father and friend that I can be. Your greatest journeys are ahead. Don't settle for anything less than the greatness that is in each of you. Thank you for being shining beacons of joy in my life. (P.S.: Don't forget about the arm-wrestle dating clause.)

Mom, you've taught me a great deal about parenthood. I took your sacrifices for granted when I was a child. It was only later in life that I realized how much you gave to Josh and me. Your love, lust for life, travel and constant learning have been the greatest gifts that you have given me. Thank you for your unconditional support. *I will love you forever*.

Dad, you provided much to me in my life, but none more important than patience and kindness. Your empathy and stoic understanding of the human condition are two skills I strive to master. I admire your passion for doing a job well (the first time), which I strive to emulate everyday. You are a rock-solid role model.

To my brother, Josh, our childhood fights, fun-filled games, and laugh attacks shaped who we are today. You are one of my closest friends, not to mention one of the coolest people I know. Don't stop doing what you love—and I promise to do the same. Thanks for being the best "bigger-little brother" a guy could ever hope for.

To James (*the* MFCEO), thank you for showing me that passion and business can coexist. Over the past 18 years, I've learned a lot from your competitive nature and shrewd business sense. Thank you for taking me under your wing, being a mentor in life and business, and for encouraging me to chase my dreams and passions.

To Brian and Cheryl, thank you for your friendship and support over the last few years. You've been great guinea pigs for the Whole Life Fitness Program. Even when worn out from Workout of the Days (WODS), unable to articulate a complaint or a compliment, you always found the energy to smile and ask for more. (T.S.E. trademark pending! LOL.)

To my Sunday Funday family and #WLFManifesto tribe, you've helped me realize that coaching is my calling. Your willingness to learn, adapt and constantly improve pushed me in more ways than you'll ever know. Your friendships, words of encouragement, and continuous support showed me that community is one of the greatest assets anyone can have and that it must be nurtured and treated with respect, love and kindness. I appreciate your courage and commitment to a better "you," one workout at a time. Thank you.

To the best book team ever: Maggie, Lucy, Mauve, Paris, Rachel, JoAnne, Margaret and Ron. With your dedication, expert advice, guidance, patience and passion for my vision, you helped make the *Whole Life Fitness Manifesto* a piece that I am truly proud to share with the world.

And to my readers and friends, online and offline, thank you for wanting the world to be nothing less than awesome.

If life is like a burpee, I'm ready and willing to make it the best WOD possible. After all, burpees condition us for one of the greatest skills in life—the ability to get back up and keep pressing forward, even when we'd rather take the path of least resistance. Don't ever stop getting up!

And yes, #BuckFurpees! Hoorah!